Case Management of

Long-Term Conditions

Principles and Practice for Nurses

Janet Snoddon
MSc, BA, SRN, SCM, DN
Deputy Director of Corporate Performance & Standards, NHS Sefton

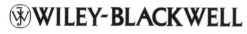

WILEY-BLACKWELL

A John Wiley & Sons, Ltd., Publication

This edition first published 2010
© 2010 Blackwell Publishing Ltd

Blackwell Publishing was acquired by John Wiley & Sons in February 2007.
Blackwell's publishing programme has been merged with Wiley's global Scientific,
Technical, and Medical business to form Wiley-Blackwell.

Registered office
John Wiley & Sons Ltd, The Atrium, Southern Gate, Chichester, West Sussex, PO19 8SQ,
United Kingdom

Editorial offices
9600 Garsington Road, Oxford, OX4 2DQ, United Kingdom
350 Main Street, Malden, MA 02148-5020, USA

For details of our global editorial offices, for customer services and for information
about how to apply for permission to reuse the copyright material in this book please
see our website at www.wiley.com/wiley-blackwell.

The right of the author to be identified as the author of this work has been asserted in
accordance with the UK Copyright, Designs and Patents Act 1988.

Library of Congress Cataloging-in-Publication Data

Snoddon, Janet.
    Case management of long-term conditions : principles and practice for nurses / Janet
Snoddon.
       p. ; cm.
    Includes bibliographical references and index.
       ISBN 978-1-4051-8005-4 (pbk. : alk. paper)   1. Chronic diseases—Nursing.
2. Chronically ill—Care.   3. Hospitals—Case management services.   I. Title.
    [DNLM: 1. Chronic Disease—nursing.   2. Case Management.   3. Long-Term
Care—methods. WY 152 S673c 2010]
    RT120.C45S657 2010
    616′.044—dc22

                                                                    2009042944

A catalogue record for this book is available from the British Library.

Set in 10/12.5 pt Palatino by MPS Limited, A Macmillan Company, Chennai, India
Printed and bound in Malaysia by KHL Printing Co Sdn Bhd

1   2010

Contents

Introduction   ix

**1 Background to the Implementation of Case Management Models for
    Chronic Long-Term Conditions within the National Health Service**   **1**

   Introduction   1
   Primary care management of long-term conditions   2
   How management approaches have been developed   3
   Developing and delivering care   4
   Future of care   5
   The impact and cost of chronic disease   6
   Identifying patients who require case management   7
   National guidelines and evidence-based practice   8
   Embedding evidence in practice   8
   Making progress in the management of chronic conditions   9
   Modernising care in the National Health Service   10
   Developing case management and care delivery   10
   Case management in the National Health Service   11
   Promotion of self-management and self-care   13
   Partnerships and expectations   13
   Conclusion   15
   References   15

2 Case Management Models: Nationally and Internationally   **18**

   Introduction   18
   The context for case management in the NHS   20
   Impact of managed care models   21
   International models of care reviewed   22
   The Alaskan Medical Service   22
   Kaiser Permanente (North California)   24
   Group Health Cooperative (Seattle, Washington)   25
   HealthPartners (Minnesota)   25
   Touchpoint Health Plan (Wisconsin)   26
   Anthem Blue Cross and Blue Shield (Connecticut)   26
   UnitedHealth Europe Evercare   26
   Amsterdam HealthCare System (the Netherlands)   27
   Outcome intervention model (New Zealand)   28
   National model of chronic disease prevention and control (Australia)   28

Guided Care (United States)   28
PACE (United States)   28
Veterans Affairs (Unites States)   29
Improving Chronic Illness Care (Seattle)   29
Expanded Chronic Care Model (Canada)   29
Pfizer (United States)   29
Green Ribbon Health: Medicare in health support (Florida)   30
What do these models provide?   30
Models in use in England   30
Care management in social care   32
Case management models in the NHS   32
Joint NHS and social care   36
Data for case management   38
Evaluation   38
Conclusion   40
References   41

3 **Competencies for Managing Long-Term Conditions**   **43**

Introduction   43
Development of the competency framework   44
What the competencies are expected to deliver   46
The competencies: what are they?   46
Domain A: advanced clinical nursing practice   47
Domain B: leading complex care co-ordination   49
Domain C: proactively manage complex long-term conditions   52
Domain D: managing cognitive impairment and mental well-being   52
Domain E: supporting self-care, self-management and enabling
independence   55
Domain F: professional practice and leadership   57
Domain G: identifying high-risk people, promoting health
and preventing ill health   58
Domain H: end-of-life care   59
Domain I: interagency and partnership working   60
What the competencies aim to do   61
Developing educational models to develop competencies   62
Conclusion   64
References   64

4 **Outcomes for Patients – Managing Complex Care**   **66**

Introduction   66
The areas of competence and deliverables for patients: Leading
complex care co-ordination   66
Identifying high-risk patients, promoting health and
preventing ill health   74

Interagency and partnership working   77
Conclusion   82
References   82

5 **Outcomes for Patients – Advanced Nursing Practice**   **85**

Introduction   85
Advanced clinical nursing practice   85
Proactively manage complex long-term conditions   91
Professional practice and leadership   94
Managing care at the end of life   97
Conclusion   101
References   102

6 **Outcomes of Case Management for Social Care and Older People** **105**

Introduction   105
Policy drivers for the care of older people   105
Health and social care integration   108
Cost of care for older people   109
What do people expect in old age and how will these
services be commissioned?   111
What does case management offer to older people?   112
Integrated models of care   114
Impact of case management on older people   114
Managing resources   118
Outcomes for older people   118
Conclusions   119
References   120

7 **Outcomes for Patients – Cancer Care and End-of-Life Care** **123**

Introduction   123
Gold Standards Framework for Palliative Care   125
Integrated Cancer Care Programme   125
Preparing for the pilot programmes   127
Delivering the pilots   129
Programme outcomes   130
Case Management and ICCP   131
Case management competencies – what can/should
patients expect?   132
The real need for competencies   137
Advanced care planning   139
Preferred place of care and delivering choice programmes   140
Conclusion   140
References   142

8 **Leadership and Advancing Practice**   **144**

Introduction   144
What is leadership?   144
What does leadership provide?   145
Leadership framework in the NHS   146
Skills in leadership   147
Political understanding and functioning   148
Setting targets and delivering outcomes   148
Empowerment and influencing   149
Levels of competence   150
Other leadership frameworks   150
What does good leadership do?   153
Impact on organisations   153
Leadership in case management   154
Leadership and change   155
Leadership is in every role   156
Advanced practice   157
Prescribing   158
Advanced practice in long-term conditions   159
Conclusions   160
References   161

9 **Self-Care and Patient Outcomes**   **164**

Introduction   164
What is self-care?   164
Self-care and practitioners   167
Systems for self-care   168
Expert Patient Programme   168
Effectiveness of self-care programmes   169
Promoting self-care: staff role   170
Self-care: models   171
Self-care: the evidence base   173
Using information and technology for self-care   175
How do we engage patients in self-care?   179
Conclusions   180
References   183

10 **What Does This Mean for Patients?**   **185**

Introduction   185
Government expectations   186
What do patients want from care?   186
Reported outcomes from management of long-term conditions   187
Modernisation to enable outcomes for users of services   188

Do patients really see improvement?   188
Understanding the patient experience, how we find out?   190
Public Service Agreement targets   192
Other assessments of user/patient experiences   192
Patient-centred care   195
Allowing patients to tell their tale   195
Outcomes of care and patient experience   195
Experience in case management   197
Partnerships with patients: impact on experience   199
Quality for patients   200
Impact of the provision of information on patients'
views and outcomes   201
Conclusions   201
References   203

Index   207

Introduction

'Delivering improvements for people with long term conditions isn't just about treating illness, it's about delivering personalised, responsive, holistic care in the full context of how people want to live their lives.'

David Colin-Thome, National Director for
Primary Care [1]

This text aims to provide to all appropriate practitioners across all the professions (nurses, pharmacists, physiotherapists including social care practitioners) who might be involved in delivery of proactive case management with a practical understanding of how their knowledge and skills can be utilised to improve outcomes for people with chronic long-term conditions. The text contains some broad reflections on care and service delivery based on reviews of evidence and views from clinicians in the use of these skills and competencies to deliver improved outcomes for these clients.

Chapters 4 to 7 focus in the main on practical application of the competencies which have been developed for case managers and do not describe disease-based intervention per se; some specific issues are discussed if they link to the specific competency domains. The ability of the practitioner to make a difference to patient outcomes through the use of their skills and expertise (competence) is recognised as key to ensuring the achievement of quality and outcomes for patients.

It is clear from the NHS review [2] that the areas of care which frustrate patients most are those which rely on shared or transfer of, care. This review outlines describes the push to ensure care is designed and delivered with the patient at the centre. This is defined by the International Alliance of Patients' Organisations [3] as a "healthcare system which is designed and delivered to address the healthcare needs and preferences of patients so that healthcare is appropriate and cost effective". Proponents of case management would claim that this model of care is defined as a model of healthcare delivery based on exactly this definition. The recent publication of Supporting People with Long-Term Conditions: Commissioning for Personalised Care Planning [4] further supports the ongoing development of case management models with their focus on the patient at the centre of care development and delivery.

The importance of appropriate and effective management of patients with long-term chronic conditions cannot be underestimated and both the Department of Health and the public are expecting much from the improvements and changes outlined in the recently published review by Lord Darzi [2]. The Operating Framework for 2009/2010 [5] continues this policy guidance through its focus on care closer to home, delivery of quality and outcomes and of course the requirement to ensure choice. This text aims to enable practitioners to understand how they might use their skills and expertise to deliver the care expected and required for this particularly vulnerable and needy group of patients, and of course support the delivery of the policy imperatives.

Chapter 1 provides for the practitioner an overview of the background to case management; the idea is to provide an overview only and not an in-depth review of the policy context. Many of the recent policy and strategic areas are included as these provide an important foundation to understand the direction of travel for the provision of health and social care for those with long-term chronic conditions, particularly in England. Chapter 2 provides an overview of some models in use nationally and internationally for delivery of case management, including some initial discussion of data processes used to identify appropriate patients to include in case management. Chapter 3 provides an overview of the competencies [6] for case management and processes by which practitioners may develop and continually maintain these competencies.

Chapter 4 provides an overview of the utilisation and outcomes for patients and services of competencies for the domains of leading complex care co-ordination, interagency and partnership working, and identifying high-risk patients, promoting health and preventing ill health; the chapter aims to outline what these outcomes could mean in reality to a service user. Chapter 5 focuses on the skills and competencies used managing high-intensity users focusing on competencies relating to advanced clinical nursing practice, identifying and managing high-risk patients.

Chapter 6 focuses on improving outcomes for older people and those requiring social care support, promoting independence through the implementation of case management principals for staff in generic roles, including social workers and allied health professional [6]. Chapter 7 focuses on competencies as utilised by professionals in case management roles as they relate directly to managing patients with cancer and at the end of life. Chapter 8 focuses on leadership and advancing practice within case management and also reflects in more detail on the issue relating to data not only for identification of patients for case management but also in relation to outcomes, effectiveness and quality. Chapter 9 reviews the process for self care and the role of professionals in its delivery. This chapter also looks briefly at the need for improvements in the health decisions made by the population in relation to prevention of chronic disease and improved outcomes through self care. The effectiveness of programmes and the need of commissioners to actually commission the programmes is also discussed [7,8]. Chapter 10 attempts to bring together an overview from each chapter focusing on evaluation of care delivery and the views of patients and carers.

In writing this text the author, who is an experienced practitioner and senior National Health Service Manager and who has through practical application developed and implemented case management services, skills and competencies, has used her clinical and managerial experiences to provide a realistic outline of the use of the skills and how these skills can improve outcomes for patients. It is hoped that the text will both inform and support practitioners and enable them to develop further their skills and understanding for the benefit of patients.

References

1. Department of Health (2008). *Raising the Profile of Long Term Conditions Care: A Compendium of Information.* http://www.dh.gov.uk/prod_consum_dh/groups/dh_ digitalassets/documents/digitalasset/dh_082067.pdf (accessed on October 2009).
2. Department of Health (2008). *High Quality Care for All: NHS Next Stage Review, Final Report.* http://www.dh.gov.uk/prod_consum_dh/groups/dh_digitalassets/@dh/@ en/documents/digitalasset/dh_085828.pdf (accessed on October 2009).
3. International Alliance of Patients' Organisations (IAPO) (2007). *What is Patient-Centred Healthcare? A Review of Definitions and Principles.* http://www.patientsorganizations. org/pchreview (accessed on October 2009).
4. Department of Health (January 2009). *Supporting People with Long Term Conditions: Commissioning Personalised Care Planning. A Guide for Commissioners.* http://www. dh.gov.uk/prod_consum_dh/groups/dh_digitalassets/documents/digitalasset/dh_ 093360.pdf (accessed on October 2009).
5. Department of Health (2009). *Operating Framework 2009/2010.* http://www.dh.gov. uk/prod_consum_dh/groups/dh_digitalassets/@dh/@en/documents/digitalasset/ dh_091446.pdf (accessed on October 2009).
6. Department of Health (2006). *Caring for People with Long Term Conditions: An Education Framework for Community Matrons and Case Managers.* http://www.dh.gov.uk/prod_ consum_dh/groups/dh_digitalassets/@dh/@en/documents/digitalasset/dh_ 4134012.pdf (accessed on October 2009).
7. Dixon A (2008). *Motivation and Confidence: What Does It Take to Change Behaviour?* King's Fund. http://www.kingsfund.org.uk/applications/site_search/?term=Motivation+ and+Confidence%3A+What+Does+It+Take+to+Change+Behaviour%3F+&oldterm= Motivation+and+confidence&old_term=Motivation+and+confidence&old_instance_ id=180578&submit.x=32&submit.y=9 (accessed on October 2009).
8. Boyce T, Robertson R and Dixon A (2008). *Commissioning and Behaviour Change: Kicking the Habits. Final Report.* King's Fund. http://www.kingsfund.org.uk/applications/ site_search/?term=Commissioning+and+Behaviour+Change%3A+Kicking+the+ Habits.&oldterm=Motivation+and+Confidence%3A+What+Does+It+Take+to+Chan ge+Behaviour%3F+&old_term=Motivation+and+Confidence%3A+What+Does+It+ Take+to+Change+Behaviour%3F+&old_instance_id=180580&submit.x=23&submit. y=13 (accessed on October 2009).

Chapter 1

Background to the Implementation of Case Management Models for Chronic Long-Term Conditions within the National Health Service

Introduction

Long-term conditions are defined as those conditions that cannot be cured but can be controlled by medication and other therapies. The management of chronic long-term conditions such as diabetes, chronic obstructive pulmonary disease, arthritis and heart failure is not new; for many years, specialist teams of nurses and other professionals alongside primary care generalist practitioners, including practice nurses, have been delivering specifically focused disease management for patients with chronic conditions. It is clear from health statistics that the number of diseases that are now being managed as chronic conditions is increasing as our management abilities for diseases that were once considered life threatening have improved. The patients therefore now live longer with these conditions. However, the effect of chronic diseases on the quality of life of these patients and their carers is significant.

Improving the care provided to patients with long-term conditions has been a key priority for the National Health Service (NHS) since the development of the NHS Plan in 2000 [1] and continues as a main thread through all policy drivers to be high on the Government and Department of Health (DH) agenda. It is also clear that in the NHS in England the ongoing management of these conditions is always likely to cost much more than the elective surgical procedures. There is also an economic impact of chronic diseases on the patients and their families owing to the reduction in earning potential of the younger people who develop chronic diseases and the cost of caring. Evidence suggests that the prevalence and impact of chronic diseases are greater in areas of high deprivation, and primary care trusts (PCTs) are currently attempting to improve this by focussing on behaviour change to aid prevention in these areas. The depth of evidence of inequalities in health is currently focussing the minds of commissioners on defining service needs based on real health needs, so that the services are appropriately targeted and include the provision of health promotion and prevention of disease starting early in life, and then building on this behaviour change across age ranges.

The delivery of care for those with chronic conditions with less complex needs is now clearly focused within primary care. NHS policy sets out clear expectations on commissioners to ensure that care provision is provided nearer to patients and increasing amount of care is delivered outside the acute sector, but it must be noted that other key policy and modernisation drivers aiming to introduce market-style incentives and multiple provider models may inhibit the development of good long-term disease management. The January 2009 DH publication 'Supporting people with long-term conditions: commissioning personalised care planning' [2] clearly defines for commissioners the expectations and ongoing push from a policy perspective in relation to effective commissioning of services in both health and social care for patients with long-term conditions. Each year the operating framework provides commissioners with guidance on the areas they are expected to commission and the services they need to develop, and the recent framework [3] continues to support the push of service development for patients with long-term conditions through increasing choice, commissioning care closer to the patient and focussing on commissioning for improved clinical and patient-reported outcomes.

Primary care management of long-term conditions

Increased primary care functionality in relation to chronic disease has been developed and consolidated through the recent General Medical Services contract [4], which defines the basic outline of service within primary care, and the supporting Quality and Outcomes Framework [5], which sets clear quality targets and indicators in some key areas of chronic disease management, including clinical and organisational areas; all of these domains are set in line with known good practice. The Quality and Outcomes Framework prevalence results for 2006/2007 provide information on the prevalence of many chronic diseases within England (Table 1.1). This information has enabled primary care to define in detail the service needs of the population on a practice and locality basis. The information also allows practice to identify based on national expectations the effectiveness of screening and diagnosis within the practice population. The ability of local health commissioners to use this information intelligently to commission locally based and responsive services is a major thrust to the plans for World Class Commissioning within the NHS [29].

The outcomes for the disease or condition focused services within primary care and specialist teams have improved over the years and in many areas the care has clearly been proved excellent. The publication of National Service Frameworks (NSFs) within some of the chronic disease areas has provided some clear and evidence-based processes of care, but without some supportive processes, guidelines alone could not achieve the impact on quality of care.

Table 1.1 Quality and Outcomes Framework 2006/2007 Prevalence Counts (Department of Health Data)

Long-term conditions	Numbers affected
Coronary heart disease	1,899,000
Heart failure	420,000
Stroke and transient ischaemic attack	863,000
Hypertension	6,706,000
Diabetes	1,962,000
Chronic obstructive pulmonary disease	766,000
Epilepsy	321,000
Cancer	489,000
Severe mental health conditions	380,000
Asthma	3,100,000

How management approaches have been developed

Many of the developments in the quality of care for chronic diseases, particularly heart disease, chronic obstructive airways disease and diabetes, in primary care have been assisted via projects and programmes supported through phase III of the National Primary Care Collaborative [6] in which a number of primary care practices across the NHS have taken part. The development of the required knowledge, clinical skills and competencies within practitioners to enable the management of patients with these disease processes is obviously fundamental to ensuring improved outcomes for patients. It is well known that the foundation for delivery of quality care is also based on excellent teamwork between care providers across all sectors (tertiary, acute, primary and community care) and communication between all practitioners and their patients and carers. The high-level competencies for case managers [7] that were published by the DH in 2006, and that form the main focus of the later discussion within this text, reflect many of the same skills and competencies developed by specialists and generalists. It is clear from the evidence that if this higher level of competence is held by the practitioners, they can provide the process of proactive case management and therefore enable the programme of care to provide the expected improvements in outcomes and quality of life.

The development of pathways and models of care based on evidence and good practice that are shared across acute and primary care has allowed not only the ongoing development and dissemination of skills and competencies to primary care and community practitioners but also some progress with improvements in the quality of service delivery. This ongoing development of skills and competence has also enabled the level of patient complexity managed in primary care to continually increase, which has assisted in the delivery of care provision, as outlined in policy documents, in a standardised way in primary care, in line with defined patient pathways and of course good practice. These developments in care provision have effectively enabled the movement of a reasonable proportion of care out from acute settings nearer to the patient, which is clearly in line with many of the current policy require-ments including the recently published report by Lord Darzi 'High-quality care for all: NHS Next Stage Review' [8].

The long-term development of the General Medical Services contract over the past decade has also provided practices with the ability to increase capacity and to develop in their staff the specific skills and knowledge required to provide care in particular disease areas based on the health needs of their practice pop-ulation. Despite all this good work, the ability to deliver quality management for patients with more than one chronic disease or with complex health needs has not progressed to the same degree, and as is clear from the evidence of the health needs of these patients who are accessing care in increasing amounts from the NHS, this cannot continue.

Developing and delivering care

It is obvious that primary care practitioners and specialist teams, both com-munity and secondary care based, have worked hard to develop the knowl-edge, skills and competencies required to manage these chronic-disease-specific programmes of care and this has improved greatly the communication between them. However, there remains an overall view within the NHS, which is reported anecdotally by patients and carers, of lack of 'co-ordination' and 'personalisation' of care for those with more than one condition and who are at the more complex end of care need.

Nevertheless, from both the patient and the delivery perspectives, it is clear that as the population becomes older and lives longer with chronic conditions, managing patients with any of these diseases in disease-based silos, particularly when many of the patients have more than one chronic disease, is a recipe for confusion and is unsatisfactory in terms of outcomes. This silo-based process of care delivery very clearly achieves much poorer patient outcomes and lower levels of patient satisfaction. Although the care being delivered is obviously well meant and often of a high standard, the lack of personalisation does in some cases lead to less than successful outcomes for patients and their carers as the care received is often viewed as inflexible and not always based on the patients' wishes, nor does the service delivery always reflect patients' choice. The process of case management and its formalised implementation is now seen by the NHS as a potential way to improve both the outcomes and the effectiveness of care delivery for patients with multiple conditions and complex needs; this patient group is often described in policy and planning documents as 'high-intensity users'. The improved management of these patients is seen as a key process that will reduce their impact on acute services through reduction in emergency admissions.

As outlined previously, the United Kingdom has, alongside most industrialised countries, improved the management of many of the individual chronic diseases through advances in understanding of disease processes, improving non-pharmacological and pharmacological management and setting of good practice standards based on a sound evidence base. The NHS has also, through a number of projects and programmes, aimed to improve the way service is delivered through 'good practice'. A key programme to facilitate improved care models includes the implementation of the National Institute for Health and Clinical Excellence, which publishes a wide range of guidance relating to care delivery commonly known as NICE guidance. NICE guidance, either technology or intervention based, is published to provide healthcare staff, providers and commissioners with a robust review of the clinical effectiveness of treatment practices and interventions including medication appraisals. The implementation of the processes within NICE guidance, though not always popular with the public, professionals or the pharmaceutical industry, does at least provide for the first time a formalised and systematic review of treatments and interventions within the NHS.

Historically, this sort of review and evidence was not always widely or easily available within the NHS despite the work of many academic departments and clinical/research teams across universities and the NHS. A number of teams within UK academic establishments have developed processes and delivered systematic review projects over the years. One of the most established, well known and credible is the Cochrane Collaboration [9], which has defined very clearly the gold standard for processes of reviews, including guidance for the processes that should be utilised to ensure the quality and efficacy of any review. Although at one time it was claimed that very few interventions used routinely within the NHS had been subject to any robust or systematic review of efficacy or effectiveness, it is now seen as an absolutely fundamental requirement that clinical interventions and treatments provided are evaluated for clinical and cost effectiveness and that all services are now subject to appropriately robust review to ensure safe care and value for money. The NHS Centre for Reviews and Dissemination is also a key player in the area of practice and service review and dissemination of learning.

Future of care

The major review of funding completed by Derek Wanless and published in April 2002 [10] provided a number of potential 'scenarios' for the funding of health care up to 2022/2023. The scenarios presented were based on assumptions regarding the effectiveness of the NHS performance and the health status of the population. The report clearly outlines the need for the NHS to improve dramatically the quality and outcomes of care provision as without these improvements any increase in funding would be, in the main, ineffective and care would gradually become more and more unaffordable. For more than a decade, the NHS has undergone a programme of reform and modernisation in which the NHS budget in England has trebled to reach £93.6 billion, in Northern Ireland there has been a 35% increase in budget and in Scotland the budget has increased by 76% since 1999 [11]. This level of investment has clearly delivered some quality and service improvements, but still there remain concerns regarding the quality and effectiveness of some of the programmes of care for the most vulnerable and, of course, for those with the most complex needs, in particular with chronic conditions.

The investment has accompanied much reorganisation with healthcare delivery including improved commissioning processes via PCTs, payment by results (PBR), world class commissioning, practice-based commissioning (PBC) and foundation trusts. All of these changes are focused on delivering an NHS improvement plan [30] through the implementation of a 'patient-led NHS', in which money follows patients and commissioning decisions are based on clearly defined health needs [12]. The NHS is trying through modernisation to:

- Shift care away from relatively expensive inpatient care to community-based diagnosis and management,
- Achieve economies of scale through integration of institutions,
- Control clinical profligacy through clinical guidelines and evidence-based practice,
- Substitute expensive doctors with less expensive professionals,
- Implement provider performance monitoring to improve quality and accountability.

The impact and cost of chronic disease

It has been estimated that in Britain 17.5 million adults may be living with a chronic disease and that 6 in 10 adults in the household population report some form of chronic health problem [13]. The number of people over 65 is projected to increase across the United Kingdom by between 18% and 23% and the number of people aged 85 or over is projected to rise by nearly 75% by 2025 [11], and it is also likely that 75% of people over the age of 75 are or will be suffering from some form of chronic health problem. The fact is that older people are the main users of the NHS, and although they form only about one-fifth of the population, it is known that they occupy two-third of general and acute beds within NHS hospitals [14]. This activity and cost pressure is not just on the NHS; even the local authorities spent nearly half of their social service budget during 1999/2000 on older people (NSF for older people) [15]. A key target for local authorities is to increase the number of people living independently in their areas. The processes used are direct payments, which can empower clients to choose the care they desire, and improved services, which enable independence with availability of equipment and telecare and care management (assessment and care planning). The requirement for local authorities and the NHS to work in partnership to deliver services is also fundamental to enabling independence.

The figures for chronic diseases in the United Kingdom, reflected in World Health Organisation data across the industrialised world, highlight that some 75% of the total population reports having one chronic condition and 50% reports having two or more conditions [13]. The figures describe very clearly the size of the problem facing the NHS both now and in the future.

Identifying patients who require case management

The development of a process to identify patients who are in need or at risk of readmissions or who require specific service delivery has been carried out in a number of ways across the NHS over the years. The literature review of predictive risk processes by the King's Fund and their partners outlines the rationale for predictive modelling and the successes and failures of some of the processes used [16]. This review concludes that measurement of risk is extremely important and that good predictive models must be adaptable to the context, must be statistically valid and must contain sufficient variables; currently, concurrent modelling is seen as most accurate, but this may change as we utilise more intelligent data. The variables used in the models are seen as interdependent. It is clear from this review that socio-economic data alone have low predictive power, but the power increases when they are linked to other variables including diagnostics, clinical data and pharmacy data. The development of predictive tools, such as the Patients at Risk of Re-hospitalisation (PARR) [17] tool and Dr Foster Intelligence's High-impact User Manager (HUM) system, to assist in the identification of patients at high risk has provided some support to organisations trying to implement case management. The combined PARR tool is an algorithm that merges a number of data variables, including hospital episode statistics (HES) and community data, to identify effectively the patients at high risk of re-admission. The PARR tool [18] developed by a collaboration of the King's Fund, New York Centre for Health and Public Service Research and Health Dialog Solutions has provided to PCTs across England an intelligent analytical tool. The tool has been used successfully in many organisations for identifying and targeting care for patients at the highest risk. The tool has been further developed to provide information on needs across the full chronic disease continuum.

The combined predictive model has provided a process through which organisation have been able to tailor interventions to the needs of the patients and match the expected outcomes. This model enables organisations to focus efforts on areas of need across the full spectrum of the risk pyramid. The PARR tool provides well-validated statistical information on patients and their level of risk in relation to service usage. The DH has also supported the development of predictive tools and provided a data toolkit [19] that aims to assist health and social care partners in understanding the health impact of chronic diseases on their populations. The accessibility of 'intelligent' information allows the organisations to understand which diseases are having the greatest negative impact on the local population and where. The information can then be utilised to inform commissioning decisions, allowing improved local planning and targeted service delivery to improve outcomes and reduce health inequalities. It should also be noted that though predictive tools based on analysis of data are effective, identification by clinicians and practitioners based on their knowledge of patients has also been used and found to be reasonably effective in outcomes.

National guidelines and evidence-based practice

The development for the NHS of the NSFs [15] for diabetes, mental health, coronary heart disease and older people during the late 1990s initiated standardised, evidence-based care programmes/pathways for the long-term conditions and care groups. The NSFs were developed for clinical areas of high population exposure and outlined care pathways based on robust evidence with proven efficacy. The publication of the NSFs provided for the first time some clear national targets for quality standards and outcomes within service provision and delivery targets to facilitate and enable service improvements across the NHS. Despite these targets, implementation has in some areas been patchy, with greater levels of success in those areas for which implementation funding followed targets. However, the delivery targets within NSFs have provided a framework on which commissioners and providers, including clinicians, have been able to influence improvements and changes in service delivery. The targets within NSFs have in the main been focused on increasing access to service pathways modelled on good practice, by ensuring that standardisation of care is implemented to improve both access to care and the quality of its delivery. The development and implementation of evidence-based guidelines like NICE guidance and NSFs into care delivery is heavily dependent on the credibility of the guidelines and the organisation/group that produces this information. Despite well-disseminated guidelines within the NHS, there remain some areas in which full implementation is challenging.

Embedding evidence in practice

The Institute for Healthcare Improvement in the United States would argue that a delivery infrastructure is required for embedding evidence-based guidance into practice. The areas that they advise as good practice would not be a surprise to anyone working in clinical care as these are seen as absolutely essential to enable effective implementation. The supporting processes can be described simply as:

- Find the guidance,
- Encourage providers to take part in the process,
- Check what you currently do,
- Customise to local needs as appropriate,

- Use simple flow charts and checklists to ensure full understanding,
- Review both effectiveness of delivery and the guideline.

The evaluative process outlined also allows for identification of barriers to implementation, which should then, in theory, allow planning for any other implementation to manage these issues in advance. It is clear from reviews of effective guideline implementation that there are a number of other key principles to enable embedding of guidelines, which are in many ways common sense. Effective implementation will obviously rely on the clinical engagement and the involvement early in the process of those likely to be most negative; winning their hearts and minds will most definitely assist the process. It is also clear from what we know about delivery of project management that implementation of a guideline would be assisted by project management processes. These project management processes allow for clear planning and timescales and also for identification of pressures and problems that might delay or prevent implementation. This does not mean that every guideline needs full project management methodology, but the principles of understanding the aim, knowing the journey and supporting the trajectory of the journey would dramatically improve implementation. Within the NHS we rely, in many instances, on dissemination of guidance to practitioners and their ability and commitment to implementation, and whilst for some this will be an easy and effective process, for others it most definitely is not the most appropriate way to support delivery. All NHS organisations are required to declare compliance with the Standards for Better Health to evidence how they provide assurance of dissemination and implementation of national clinical guidelines and how they develop and implement local clinical pathways as part of world class commissioning.

Making progress in the management of chronic conditions

Improvements in management of chronic conditions are clearly evidenced by the fact that mortality from heart disease had fallen across the United Kingdom by 27% between 1996/1997 and 2001/2003; this is alongside a reduction in death rates from cancer in the under 75 group by 12% in the 6 years up to 2005 [20]. There is therefore evidence of increasing life expectancy of many patients with long-term conditions. The improvements in how the NHS manages these conditions have of course increased the numbers in the population living with long-term conditions across many of the disease areas. Many diseases that were considered life threatening in the past have now become chronic. An added element for the NHS in the delivery of care for patients with long-term conditions is the impact of health inequalities in these disease groups across large portions of the population. The latest information produced by national reports from the results of the Quality and Outcomes Framework in primary care [21] highlights the levels of difference in terms of both access to care and outcomes for many of the chronic diseases in areas with high levels of deprivation. The prevalence of long-term conditions varies across regions, with the England average on 33.2% with a variation of between 20% in the bottom quintile and 37–48% in the top quintile [22]. A number of factors, including age, socio-economic status and lifestyle choices, are suggested as reasons for this variation. The modernisation agenda for the NHS through PCTs aims to focus the commissioners onto potential ways to improve the health of their local population, reduce health inequalities and improve outcomes for patients.

Modernising care in the National Health Service

The NHS Reviews, like the Darzi Review [8], and modernisation plans are clearly focused on commissioning and providing services that improve the quality of life for patients. The strap line used of 'adding life to years alongside years to life' provides a new focus for the NHS, requiring that services work to improve the quality of life for patients, particularly relevant to those living with chronic conditions. It is clearly important that all providers of care focus on both quality and outcomes within service delivery and ensure that there are choices in management approaches for patients, supported with good information to facilitate those choices. The Next Stage Review [8] clearly outlines the requirement for personalised and holistic services, which are flexible in delivery and can deliver good 'patient reporting outcomes'.

It is also estimated that 45% of those with chronic disease will suffer from more than one condition, which adds complexity to the management of their disease. This can cause major problems for patients with contradictory or confusing processes of care, as these processes could be viewed by patients as narrow and unhelpful. The anecdotal comments of patients and their carers often highlight the sometimes frustrating and confusing processes of care they receive. The key comments reported outline that poor communication, poor co-ordination and lack of information are often at the heart of the problems the patients see with the care they receive.

Developing case management and care delivery

The DH has produced, based on the chronic care models, a pyramid of care that shows risk for service use of the population [18]. Those in the low-risk sector, between 21% and 100% of the population, use less than half of the average access to care (general practioners, accident and emergency [A&E] attendances and admissions). In service delivery impact, this low-risk group will require little actual intervention but may require lifestyle and other behavioural modifications. Moderate-risk group, 6–20% of the population, uses 1.8 times the average for admissions, 2.2 times the average for outpatient encounters and 1.5 times the average for A&E attendance. The moderate-risk group will require what is described as information therapy: support and information for self-care. High-risk group, equating to 0.5–5% of population, access 5.4 times the average hospital admissions, 4 times the average outpatients encounters and almost 3 times the average A&E attendances. The high-risk group needs proactive disease management at a moderate intensity. Then there is the very high risk population that forms for most organisations 0.5% of the population. This group uses more than 18 times the average for admissions, 6 times the average for outpatient contacts and 9 times the average for A&E attendances. This is very clearly the group for which care management would be the most effective.

Case management, which is seen as an option for management that can improve the process of care, can be described as a process of proactive management of patients with chronic diseases. In the main, the programme is implemented for patients with complex health needs and focuses on the use of practitioner skills, which facilitate and enable patient-centred and holistic care. The key to the process is to manage across all care environments through proactive interventions and planned programmes of care, which allow flexibility and are also focused on monitoring how the patient's condition is progressing and recognising early signs of change and deterioration. The key processes within the case management programmes in the United States are described as care orchestration, communication, acting as a champion or advocate, high-level clinical skills and acting as a coach [23]. All of these processes or skills are seen as fundamental to enabling the proactive model of care and achieving good outcomes for patients and their carers.

Case management as an advanced clinical role, for mainly nurses, has been developed in the United States. The process is fundamental to the provision of care under many of the United States healthcare providers (managed care organisations), and their aim is to programme and orchestrate care in a managed and outcome-focused way. The model has provided for the United States a cost benefit in terms of reduced admissions and improved cost effectiveness of care; these are of course essential to ensure cost control and reduction within the United States healthcare model.

Case management in the National Health Service

The implementation of case management as a process for the NHS has been encouraged via the DH through support to PCTs pilots of case management models across England. The key pilot for case management was based on the United States models including Evercare programme via the UnitedHealth Group and was completed on 10 sites across the United Kingdom. The work with UnitedHealth Europe started in 1987 and a final report into the pilots was published in February 2005 [23]. The report described some key successes including increased skills and confidence within the nurses trained through the programme, high levels of patient and carer satisfaction and a reduction in hospital admissions in the biggest group of patients in the programme. However, the researchers were unable to confirm whether the latter was regression to mean or the impact of the interventions.

The DH was clearly impressed by the outcomes evidence from the pilot and set targets for each strategic health authority for the implementation of case management roles in practice. The effectiveness of these roles was measured as a Public Service Agreement (PSA) target on the basis of reduction in emergency bed days used. The PSA for long-term conditions was based on the following target: 'to improve health outcomes for people with long-term condition by offering a personalised care plan for vulnerable people at highest risk and to reduce emergency bed-days by 5% by 2008 through improved care in primary care and community settings for people with long-term conditions.' A PSA target for staff working in community matron roles, providing case management in primary or community care settings for people with complex long-term conditions and high-intensity needs, was set at 3000 nationally based on the population, with each PCT receiving an individual target.

The department has adopted the Kaiser model that stratifies people with long-term conditions into three levels. At level 1 is supportive self-care, aimed at working in collaboration with patients and carers to assist them in developing their abilities to care for themselves. Level 2 is disease-specific care management, providing responsive care for people with complex single needs through multidisciplinary teams and the disease-specific protocols such as NSFs etc. Level 3 is the identification of the most vulnerable people with highly complex multiple long-term conditions and use of case management approaches to anticipate, co-ordinate and join up health and social care.

The development of case management models to deliver improved health outcomes was therefore seen as a wise investment and as an effective way to support delivery of the PSA targets. The founding principle these targets were based on was fairly clear evidence that despite the improvements in disease-specific care through implementation of NSFs, problems persist for patients with multiple long-term conditions, leading to poor health outcomes and frequent admissions. Meeting the different elements of the PSA target required significant changes to the traditional patterns of service delivery.

The NHS data [13] show that 80% of general practitioner consultations are for patients with chronic diseases. Two-thirds of patients admitted as medical emergencies have exacerbation of chronic disease or have a chronic disease and 60% of hospital bed-days are used by patients with chronic conditions. It is also clear from these data that patients with one or more conditions make much higher use of healthcare services, e.g. the 15% of people with three or more problems account for almost 30% of inpatient days and costs for patients with more than one chronic conditions are six times higher than costs for patents with one chronic condition. These findings are no surprise to staff working in the NHS and are supported by the evidence from the United States, where it has been shown that people with chronic conditions consume about 78% of all healthcare spending [13].

The DH has supported the formal development of a case management competencies framework and a supporting educational framework [7] via an academic programme to help case managers develop the set of competencies that are required for providing effective care. The implementation of case management model is also fundamental to organising care around the needs of patients and nearer to where they live, promoting self-care models and improving outcomes of care. It should be noted that in addition to this model of care delivery, there has been an increased recognition of the need to focus on prevention of long-term conditions through lifestyle changes, increase early diagnosis through access to effective screening programmes, improve personal abilities to self-care through robust education on diagnosis and facilitate the delivery of choice.

Promotion of self-management and self-care

The Expert Patients Programme [31] is one of the initiatives aimed at supporting and enabling patients to make informed choices and improving their abilities to self-care. All of these are fundamental principles in delivering improved health outcomes and processes for the management of long-term conditions. NHS targets to enable patients to take personal responsibility for their own well-being and also provide ongoing support for self-care. This will result in delivery of improved outcomes for health through compliance and concordance and an increasing recognition within patients of the importance of lifestyle choices in the ongoing progress of chronic diseases [11]. The principle of personal responsibility is underwritten in the NHS Constitution [25]. The current published constitution outlines for the first time the rights and responsibilities of the public and staff. It not only outlines the need for all users of the NHS to accept their personal responsibilities for working in partnership with care providers but also clearly outlines what a patient can expect from the NHS and its staff.

Partnerships and expectations

There is also a clear recognition that the partnership of care delivery across health and social care is fundamental to managing long-term care in the future, as without collaboration and integration, care delivery will be fundamentally flawed. Health and social care systems must therefore consider the effect of the aging population on the demands for resources.

> The best care and support is delivered by professionals working together as part of teams to meet the needs of communities, groups and individuals. There are huge benefits for everyone – NHS, local authorities, third sector, but most of all for all of those people whose lives can be transformed by being given the support that's right for them.
>
> David Behan, Director General for Social Care [22]

It is also clear that, in future, the expectation of commissioners of service will be that service will be delivered through a patient at the centre of care programme [12] and in a co-ordinated and integrated way. In the longer term, commissioners will commission based on patient pathways, which have safe and effective handovers of care responsibility, with proven patient outcomes and delivery nearer to the patients' home. The guidance provided to commissioners within 'Supporting people with long-term conditions: commissioning personalised care planning' [2] clearly outlines the expectations to embed personalised care planning within all health and social care economies. The document provides a clear definition of what personalised care planning should include, the benefits and what it means for the commissioners. The concept is that commissioning patient-centred services will enable improved outcomes for patients through increased service integration and partnerships, improved service user satisfaction, improved efficiency, promotion of independence and choice and reduction in health inequalities through standardised approaches to care.

The NHS White Paper 'Our Health, Our Care, Our Say' [26] and the policy document that followed it clearly outlines the need for the health and social care professionals to work together to deliver 'joined up' services which utilise a holistic view of the needs of individual patients and provide care which ensures quality of care and outcomes. It is also clear from some service reviews in local areas that recognition of the strengths of the care workforce and some development in their skills to enable delivery of ongoing review and supervision of disease management (recording of blood pressure, blood sugar etc within set parameters) could improve outcomes, provide early recognition of deterioration and increase management processes and thereby reduce emergency admissions.

The implementation and delivery of the ongoing modernisation agenda within the NHS clearly defines new and advanced roles for all professionals, alongside the plans and reports already in place, for example those outlined in many policy and strategic papers from the Chief Nursing Officer and other key leaders within the NHS [27,28]. Implementation of case management models and processes is just one of the many new roles required of healthcare professionals to enable these modernisation plans to be delivered. Healthcare provisions and roles across the world are changing constantly to enable the delivery of care based on health needs and improvement in patient outcomes.

The NHS has since its inception constantly striven to improve care quality and access to care. It has tried to deliver this through quality leadership and encouragement of innovation. The NHS Plan published in 2000 provided for all involved in care opportunities to reinvigorate and modernise care delivery. The development of processes for improved management of chronic disease care is just one area in which the opportunities are beginning to be realised.

Across the NHS, provider organisations and their partners (social care and the voluntary sector) are busily developing service to manage and support this patient group. Each of these organisations is working to manage the following key issues:

- Recruitment, education and training of the workforce,
- Targeting patients: how to identify those who will gain the most benefit,
- Processes and operational tools,
- Interface working and referral processes,
- Information and data management.

This remainder of this text attempts to review how these issues may be or are being managed and how case management can and is making a real difference to the health and social well-being of these patients.

Conclusion

It is apparent that all policy drivers in health and social care are pointing to the need to modernise care delivery. The ability of society to deliver the health and social care needs, both now and in the future, is dependent on this modernisation. The needs of the population in relation to care are increasing owing to lack of improved health behaviours, prevention and improved management of chronic conditions including self-management; therefore, modernisation of service delivery is absolutely essential. Since we now recognise the increasing burden of chronic long-term conditions on the society, this will remain the key focus for service delivery. The enormity of the impact on individuals and society of these disease processes is now well recognised as is the fact that we must prevent these disease from occurring and manage them when diagnosed. If these actions can be implemented effectively, patients/service users are more likely to live longer and healthier lives. The implementation of the recommendations within the 'Darzi Review' alongside other policy recommendations will probably enable new models of care, which are indeed focused on the personal needs and views of the population.

References

1. Department of Health (2000). *The NHS Plan*. http://www.dh.gov.uk/prod_consum_dh/groups/dh_digitalassets/@dh/@en/documents/digitalasset/dh_4055783.pdf (accessed on October 2009).
2. Department of Health (2009). *Supporting People with Long Term Conditions: Commissioning Personalised Care Planning. A Guide for Commissioners*. http://www.dh.gov.uk/en/Publicationsandstatistics/Publications/PublicationsPolicyAndGuidance/DH_093354 (accessed on October 2009).
3. Department of Health (2009). *High Quality Care for All: Operating Framework for the NHS 2009/2010*. http://www.dh.gov.uk/prod_consum_dh/groups/dh_digitalassets/@dh/@en/documents/digitalasset/dh_091446.pdf (accessed on October 2009).

4. Department of Health (April 2004). *General Medical Services Contract.* http://www. dh.gov.uk/en/Healthcare/Primarycare/Primarycarecontracting/GMS/DH_ 4125638 (accessed on October 2009).

5. Department of Health (April 2006/2007). *Quality & Outcomes Framework.* http://www. dh.gov.uk/prod_consum_dh/groups/dh_digitalassets/@dh/@en/documents/ digitalasset/dh_4088693.pdf (accessed on October 2009).

6. National Collaborating Centre for Chronic Conditions (2004). *Chronic Obstructive Pulmonary Disease. National Guidelines on the Management of Chronic Obstructive Pulmonary Disease in Adults in Primary and Secondary Care.* http://guidance.nice.org. uk/CG12 (accessed on October 2009).

7. Department of Health (2006). *Caring for People with Long Term Conditions: An Education Framework for Community Matrons and Case Managers.* http://www.dh.gov.uk/ prod_consum_dh/groups/dh_digitalassets/@dh/@en/documents/digitalasset/ dh_4118102.pdf (accessed on October 2009).

8. Department of Health (2008). *High Quality Care for All: NHS Next Stage Review Final Report.* http://www.dh.gov.uk/prod_consum_dh/groups/dh_digitalassets/@dh/@en/ documents/digitalasset/dh_085828.pdf (accessed on October 2009).

9. Cochrane Collaboration and NHS Centre for Reviews and Dissemination. http:// cochrane.co.uk/en/index.html (accessed on October 2009).

10. Wanless D (2004). *Securing Good Health for the Whole Population.* Treasury Office. http:// www.hm-treasury.gov.uk/consult_wanless04_final.htm (accessed on October 2009).

11. Department of Health (2006). *Modernising Nursing Careers.* http://www.dh.gov.uk/ prod_consum_dh/groups/dh_digitalassets/@dh/@en/documents/digitalasset/ dh_4138757.pdf (accessed on October 2009).

12. Department of Health (2005). *Patient Led NHS.* http://www.dh.gov.uk/prod_ consum_dh/groups/dh_digitalassets/@dh/@en/documents/digitalasset/dh_ 4106507.pdf (accessed on October 2009).

13. Department of Health (2008). *Improving Chronic Disease Management: A Compendium of Information.* http://www.dh.gov.uk/prod_consum_dh/groups/dh_digitalassets/ documents/digitalasset/dh_082067.pdf (accessed on October 2009).

14. 2006 UK National Audit Office. http://www.nao.org.uk/publications.aspx (accessed on October 2009).

15. National Service Frameworks Diabetes, Mental Health, Older People, Children. http:// www.dh.gov.uk/en/publicationsandstatistics/index.htm (accessed on October 2009).

16. King's Fund, NHS Modernisation Agency, Health Dialog and New York University (2006). *Predictive Risk Project Literature Review.* http://www.kingsfund.org.uk/ applications/site_search/?term=Predictive+risk+project+literature+review &searchreferer_id=0&searchreferer_url=%2Fapplications%2Fsite_search%2Findex. rm&submit.x=16&submit.y=12

17. King's Fund, Health Dialog Analytic Solutions and New York University Center for Health and Public Service Research September (2005). *Case Finding Algorithm for Patients at Risk of Re-Hospitalisation.* http://www.kingsfund.org.uk/applications/site_ search/?term=Case+Finding+Algorithm+for+Patients+at+Risk+of+Re-Hospitalisation. &searchreferer_id=0&searchreferer_url=%2Fapplications%2Fsite_search%2Findex. rm&submit.x=22&submit.y=9

18. Health Dialog (June 2006). *Combined Predictive Model: Executive Summary of Interim Results.* http://www.kingsfund.org.uk/applications/site_search/?term=Combine+ Predictive+Model%3A+Executive+Summary+of+Interim+Results.&searchrefere r_id=0&searchreferer_url=%2Fapplications%2Fsite_search%2Findex.rm&submit. x=16&submit.y=10

19. Department of Health (2009). *Disease Management Information Toolkit (DMIT)*. http://www.dh.gov.uk/prod_consum_dh/groups/dh_digitalassets/documents/ digitalasset/dh_074921.pdf and http://www.dh.gov.uk/prod_consum_dh/groups/ dh_digitalassets/documents/digitalasset/dh_074922.pdf (accessed on October 2009).

20. Department of Health (2005). *Supporting People with Long Term Conditions: Liberating the Talents of Nurses Who Care for People with Long Term Conditions*. http://www. dh.gov.uk/prod_consum_dh/groups/dh_digitalassets/@dh/@en/documents/ digitalasset/dh_4102498.pdf (accessed on October 2009).

21. Department of Health (2008). *Quality and Outcomes Framework Report*. http://www. dh.gov.uk/prod_consum_dh/groups/dh_digitalassets/@dh/@en/documents/ digitalasset/dh_4088693.pdf

22. Department of Health (2008). *Raising the Profile of Long Term Conditions Care: A Compendium of Information*. http://www.kingsfund.org.uk/applications/site_search? term=Combined+Predictive+Model%3A+Executive+Summary+of+Interim+Results. &searchreferer_id=0&searchreferer_url=%2Fapplications%2Fsite_search%2Findex. rm&submit.x=16&submit.y=10

23. UnitedHealth Europe (February 2005). *Assessment of the Evercare Programme in England 2003–2004*. http://www.dh.gov.uk/prod_consum_dh/groups/dh_digitalassets/@dh/ @en/documents/digitalasset/dh_4114224.pdf (accessed on October 2009).

24. Department of Health (2006). *Public Sector Agreements*. http://www.hm-treasury.gov. uk/pbr_csr07_psaindex.htm (accessed on October 2009).

25. Department of Health (2009). *NHS Constitution*. http://www.dh.gov.uk/prod_ consum_dh/groups/dh_digitalassets/documents/digitalasset/dh_093442.pdf (accessed on October 2009).

26. Department of Health (2006). *Our Health, Our Care, Our Say: NHS White Paper*. http://www.dh.gov.uk/prod_consum_dh/groups/dh_digitalassets/@dh/@en/ documents/digitalasset/dh_4127459.pdf (accessed on October 2009).

27. Department of Health (2002). *Liberating the Talents: Helping Primary Care Trusts and Nurses Deliver the NHS Plan* . http://www.dh.gov.uk/prod_consum_dh/groups/ dh_digitalassets/@dh/@en/documents/digitalasset/dh_4076250.pdf (accessed on October 2009).

28. Department of Health. *The Chief Nursing Officers '10 Key Roles'*. http://www.dh.gov. uk/prod_consum_dh/groups/dh_digitalassets/@dh/@en/documents/digitalasset/ dh_4101739.pdf (accessed on October 2009).

29. Department of Health (2008). *World Class Commissioning*. http://www.dh.gov.uk/ prod_consum_dh/groups/dh_digitalassets/documents/digitalasset/dh_080952.pdf (accessed on October 2009).

30. Department of Health (2004). *NHS Improvement Plan*. http://www.dh.gov.uk/prod_ consum_dh/groups/dh_digitalassets/@dh/@en/documents/digitalasset/dh_ 4084522.pdf (accessed on October 2009).

31. Department of Health (2001). *The Expert Patient Programme: A New Approach to Chronic Disease Management*. http://www.dh.gov.uk/prod_consum_dh/groups/ dh_digitalassets/@dh/@en/documents/digitalasset/dh_4018578.pdf (accessed on October 2009).

Chapter 2
Case Management Models: Nationally and Internationally

Introduction

Health care within the United States probably has the longest history of implementation of case management models through managed care organisations; the National Health Service (NHS) staff would, however, argue that they already have delivered many of the criteria within case management programmes without the development of managed care models. Social care colleagues would certainly hold the view that the implementation of case management to support people with complex social support needs is well established and has been in place for many years since the Community Care Act 1990. Despite this, the fact remains that the data on the ever increasing rates of emergency admissions to acute care, increasing access to general practitioner care by patients with chronic conditions and the anecdotal views of patients and carers would provide a different response to this view that the NHS and social care partners already do case management. The evidence would argue that if this is the case, then it is definitely not done well. Given the enormous burden of ill-health both individually and on health and social care services, any sharing of learning from effective models of care must be welcomed with open arms.

There are different views within the NHS on the appropriateness of transferring models of care from the United States to the United Kingdom. In the report from the King's Fund in 2001 'US Managed Care and PCTs: Lessons to a Small Island from a Lost Continent' [1], these views are discussed and debated in some detail. The report, which was published early in the development of Primary Care Trusts (PCTs) in the NHS and around the time the NHS was developing its projects in relation to managed care, describes the reasoning behind the move of the UK government towards progressive regulation and more overt management of clinical care. This ongoing 'modernisation' is seen as a process that is converging the UK and US healthcare systems. Although the report clearly describes the difficulties in matching the diverse and plural environment of US health care with the UK system, it does clearly recognise that the similarity in direction of travel in health care in the United States and United Kingdom is driven by the rising healthcare costs and the need to improve health outcomes and accountability. Those in the NHS would claim that the NHS has always been very closely managed centrally as the universal nature of provision has always required central policy to enable delivery, whereas the perception of level of 'management of care' within the US system is dependent on the perspective of the viewer. The development of 'managed care' in organisations has grown up from a system of very low levels of central control, which of course effects how the 'managed care' process is perceived.

The US healthcare environment is often seen as well funded, and yet it is not able to supply universal access. It is also subject to large degree of market pressures, competition, shaping by powerful stakeholders and, in the main, largely decentralised. In the United States, 87% of the population has health insurance via the government or privately but 13% remains uninsured and therefore not able to access universal health care. Although a Whitehall-directed, state-run bureaucratic environment of health care in the United Kingdom is quite different from that in the United States, there have been a number of policy changes to shift the balance of power from the centre to local NHS organisations. It could be argued that PCTs are the centre of this, with the responsibility for 75% of NHS resources allotted to their organisations, whose key function is to commission primary and secondary care to their registered populations. Alongside commissioning they also have the responsibility of improving the health of local people in partnership with the community and local authorities. These models are in some ways fairly similar to many managed care organisations within the United States, though PCTs clearly have the additional requirements of improving population health and working in partnership with local authorities. A major strength of the NHS is that it is seen to have developed in a social contract model different from the US healthcare system and therefore has a different set of values and assumptions, which are highly valued by the users.

The definition of managed care in the United States is an integrated system that manages the delivery of comprehensive healthcare services for an enrolled population. Rather than simply providing or paying for them, services are provided by providers who are contracted to the organisation, characteristics that are similar to those of the current functions within a PCT. Care is managed within this system through utilisation management (practice populations and partners of service use), capitation, risk sharing and primary care gatekeeper models for access. Some of these are also evident with the current PCT arrangements. In the United Kingdom, the primary care model, which is often seen as a strong and effective model of health care, provides a dedicated, personalised and universal service with strong community nursing support and is a service model not delivered in other countries. This is a model that is popular with users and many healthcare systems are covetous of this. Many within the NHS would argue that this effective and popular system should be strengthened with greater skill mix and use of a broader range of professionals.

Within the US healthcare system of managed care, rigorous control of clinical actions through particularly regular peer review of clinical care is fundamental to the process. Criteria for closely managing performance of interventions are clearly outlined and deviation from these is challenged. This means that there is much greater degree of clinical control in structured managed care model.

In the Unites States, the generic model of care 'chronic care model' has gained much support and underpins many of the approaches discussed in this chapter. Models of case management have been developed in a number of managed care organisations (health maintenance organisations) within the United States, but models of chronic disease management also exist in many of the countries within the European Union. There is therefore much to learn from these countries, but we must focus on the external or specific influences which may affect levels of success and which may therefore mean that there are differences in outcomes between other countries' healthcare systems and the NHS. However, the United States models of managed care organisations offering comprehensive health care for defined populations, with incentives to manage care proactively, do appear to have achieved some striking improvements, which we will review later in this chapter.

The context for case management in the NHS

The Department of Health (DH) reviewed a number of these models and piloted in 18 PCTs some of these care models under the leadership of the NHS Modernisation Agency. Although the major push for the formal pilot programme was based on the Evercare, Kaiser and Pfizer models of care, a number of organisations were supported to pilot other models and to develop 'anglicised' versions of case management models to deliver locally. This flexibility of implementation was utilised to allow local services to be developed to reflect local health needs. It must also be recognised that service provision within the United Kingdom is in many ways different from that provided in other counties and in particular within the United States. Clearly, the social services provided by local authorities are unusual in many of these other care provision models. Despite some differences, the ongoing development of PCTs does appear to be moving towards processes similar to those delivered through managed care organisations in the United States in that both are receiving capitation-based funding to provide a full range of services for all patients.

To enable a more detailed understanding of the effectiveness of care models, we need to be aware of the environment in which those services are delivered. It is clear from reviews that there is no direct comparison between the US and UK systems as the US systems are not nationally available provisions. The development of services in the US system will be heavily influenced by local influences, for example the response to cost by funders of care and consumer pressure. This is totally different to the NHS, where in the main, developments and changes are led by central government policy. Having said this, it is also clear, as reflected earlier, that the recent development of PCTs within England is starting to provide a model of organisation broadly similar to managed care models of the United States.

Spending on health care within the United States is the highest in the world, and yet it is known that 18% of the population has no form of health insurance and millions of people are under-insured. The situation is that approximately 90% of Americans with employer-funded health care access their care through a managed care organisation, which receives a 'capitated' payment for each person enrolled and is then responsible for the care of that person [2]. The number of managed care organisations increased rapidly between the 1980s and 1990s. This growth was largely in response to escalating healthcare costs, and by the late 1990s a substantial proportion of physicians were members of one or more organisations. These organisations are insurance based but may be run as 'for-profit' or 'not-for-profit' organisations. Many of the organisations are 'not-for-profit'. There is significant competition between them, which over the years has forced down costs in terms of both premiums and profitability, leading many of the organisations to restrict benefits and start a move towards more tightly managed care.

Impact of managed care models

The processes of managed care did, in the first instance, increase administrative costs and reduce patient choice and clinical autonomy and income. These restrictions unsurprisingly led to a backlash from a number of quarters and to a loosening of some controls. Reviews of the way these organisations manage and develop highlight that market pressures and incentives have changed the focus of organisations through a clear alignment of objectives for clinicians and managers. Within the United States, healthcare organisations constantly review the views and attitudes of consumers of care in relation to care provision and effectiveness (cost and outcome) as they need to constantly ensure that the customer is satisfied to maintain market share.

Improvement of healthcare quality and outcomes was another reason for the managed care organisations to use their purchasing power to commission and ensure the provision of better services for their patients. The evidence is that most of the efforts have been focused on chronic conditions because they are widespread in the population, costly (highest health cost is on managing these conditions), responsible for the greatest impact on the population (70% of deaths are related to these disease groups) and because there is sound evidence for many of the interventions for these diseases [2].

International models of care reviewed

Organisation and location	Models
Alaskan Medical Service	Not-for-profit case management
Kaiser Permanente, North California	Not-for-profit case management with stratification
Group Health Cooperative, Seattle	Not-for-profit, no stratification process, IT-base interactive health care
HealthPartners, Minnesota	Consumer-governed case management by telephone
Touchpoint Health Plan, Wisconsin	For-profit case managed in primary care
Anthem Blue Cross and Blue Shield, Connecticut	For-profit chronic disease management via primary care
United Health Care	Case management with stratification
Dutch healthcare system	Mixed insurance, long term condition (LTC) management
New Zealand outcomes-based model	Prevention and promotion
Australian chronic disease prevention and control	Prevention and promotion
Guided Care	Case management
PACE Model	Integrated service delivery
Veteran Affairs	Expanded Chronic Care Model
Robert Wood Johnson Foundation, Seattle	Improving Chronic Illness Care (ICIC)
Canada Chronic Disease Prevention Model	Expanded Chronic Care Model
Pfizer	High-risk case management supplementing current services
Green Ribbon Health: Medicare health support	Chronic conditions in the elderly

The Alaskan Medical Service [3]

The Alaskan Medical Service has been in place in Anchorage for 22 years, it provides health care to 45,000 clients across Anchorage and 50 remote villages. The model of healthcare delivery has been developed to enable a match with the native values (reflecting community, family and wider relationships) that focus on the idea that wellness is possible only with active patient and family support. There is a clear commitment to mutual aid with a balance between spiritual, mental, emotional and physical health provided with a respect for traditions including ancestry and the elders in the population. Within this model of health care the medical leadership model is thrown away to enable the delivery of a system focusing on provision of education and expertise to the customer, which enables them to meet their personal needs. This service system engages families and communities as advocates and supporters for vulnerable individuals to make changes and manage their own health. Throughout the processes the aim is to educate, advise, support and encourage, and at no time does the system blame the customer for noncompliance.

The Alaskan Service delivery is based on anticipatory care (explained as long-term thinking for a lifetime) with access to testing and interventions as locally as possible using technology as an enabler of care. But the programme also depends heavily on building long-term relationships between customers and professionals with a transfer of power and control from professionals to customers. The management process delivers proactive, pre-emptive case management and care co-ordination with a lead physician who manages the whole population over time using all the skills within the whole team. This process is underpinned by disease registers and an understanding of the health needs of the population. The teams are fully integrated and multidisciplinary across health and social care. Care and visits are planned and the impact of an individual's condition on everyone within the family is considered, and health education and self-care support are embedded in the service delivery.

It is clear that the success of the system is heavily dependent on the team focus, with mutual respect and interdependence, shared training and development and shared incentives providing ownership of programme and commitment to the ethos of care. The relationships to the system are built through primary care, and referral from primary care is for specialist intervention not acute care. All specialist care is provided via agreed protocols, pathways and service agreements, and these are delivered within clear quality parameters. Specialists are a resource for primary care and there is no handover of responsibility for care, whatever the settings care is delivered within. Primary care practitioners are at all times responsible for resource utilisation.

The keys to success in the system are standards for communication and information between practice and specialist, active development of relationships between specialists and generalists and a redistribution of procedures to the 'lowest' possible level to manage costs and shorten timescales. This requires extensive training and use of technicians, advanced nursing roles and assistants.

The Alaskan Medical System has reported success in a number of areas since the inception of its new model of provision. The healthcare provider reports that the system has improved quality and planning through the use of data and information, and that the workforce has been transformed through development and increase in recruitment and retention. There have been decreases in speciality care usage by 60%, emergency and urgent care usage by 50% and primary care usage by 20%. Patient and staff satisfaction and health outcomes have all improved and these improvements have been delivered with no comparative cost increase.

It is clear from the provider that this type of service change is radical and does take time to implement and requires cultural and behavioural changes. This is not just about processes. These changes have been about focusing on the needs of customers, not the needs of the healthcare system.

Kaiser Permanente (North California) [4]

Kaiser Permanente is a 'not-for-profit' healthcare organisation, which is a partnership between representatives of medicine and management, sharing the responsibility of organising, financing and delivering quality health care to its members (patients) on a pre-paid basis. The organisation is owned and led by doctors (doctors are shareholders), but within the management structure are two strategic and powerful nursing roles. The organisation aspires to be the world leader in improving health, and it delivers this through high-quality, affordable integrated health care. The primary care physician co-ordinates all care with specialists, arranges diagnostics, prescribes medication and therapy and arranges hospitalisation if required. The organisation includes in it enrolees those covered by Medicare (people over 65) and Medicaid (families on low incomes). There are nine Kaiser Permanente regional insurers. The organisation has exclusive contractual arrangements with Kaiser Foundation Hospitals and Permanente Medical Groups for specialist and tertiary care. The Kaiser Care Management Institute was founded in 1997 and is responsible for developing evidence-based protocols and programmes for conditions including chronic diseases. The patients are stratified into the following three levels of care [2]:

- Level 1, well-managed stable patients: 70–80% of the population;
- Level 2, unstable or have had an acute exacerbation and need care management: high-risk patients;
- Level 3, not stable or have comorbidities that require intensive case management: highly complex patients.

The organisation has changed the economics of medicine by focusing on keeping the patient healthy rather than treating the sickness through preventative care, home healthcare access via case managers, access to diagnostics and routine health appraisals. Public health and health promotion are currently significant focuses for the organisation. Physicians have a dual responsibility, that is they are required to not only manage individual patients but also to act as a steward of the resources of the organisation.

Services are provided based on vertical integration between primary and secondary care supported by an excellent information technology system and network. The keys to the success of the service are viewed by the clinicians as the integration of care, excellent leadership across primary and secondary care, excellent communication across sectors, understanding of health needs through disease registers, good incentives and bonuses for both staff and patients, quality of staff on recruitment (organisation is viewed as an employer of choice), patient education programmes delivering good health promotion and public health, use of Internet for links between medical and nursing staff and patients to enable advice and review of chronic conditions, medication reviews and renewal of prescriptions. Kaiser's own outcomes report that admission rates and length of stay for older patients in the United States are much lower than in the United Kingdom.

The organisation is a major player in the healthcare system in the United States and the need to deliver outcomes and results is fundamental to the continuation of service provision. Providers who cannot deliver the expected quality markers and outcomes will not be commissioned to provide services.

Group Health Cooperative (Seattle, Washington)

Group Health Cooperative is a consumer-governed not-for-profit healthcare system, which provides 80% of the health care to Washington, an area in which only 20% of the population has health cover. It offers a wide range of services in primary care and acute services through two of its owned hospitals. The organisation has focused in recent years on recruiting young enrolees as its population was aging. It has focused much work on developing a web-based interactive service called MyGroupHealth to enable the delivery of improved access to health care for families. The organisation is linked to the McColl Institute for Healthcare Innovation and Centre for Health Studies, which is responsible for developing for the organisation inhouse evidence-based best practice guidelines and for undertaking primary research. It is clear that this organisation in now attempting to catch up with other organisations in relation to chronic disease management through the development of a chronic care model. The chronic care model requires the following six areas of practice to make the programme work:

- self-management
- decision support (proven guidelines)
- delivery system design (clearly assign roles and tasks)
- clinical information system (disease registers)
- organisation of health care
- community (formation of alliances and partnerships with organisations)

HealthPartners (Minnesota)

This organisation is 'consumer-governed', accountable to a board drawn from members representing enrolees. Its main aim is to 'improve the health of members, patients and the community' and to be 'a trusted provider of health care, health promotion, health financing and care administration. The delivery of this vision has at its foundation the Partners for Health Programme, which emphasises population-based health targets similar to those being implemented through the NHS in England using public health planning. The organisation has worked in partnership with other managed care organisations to implement overarching clinical standards developed by the Institute for Clinical Systems Improvement.

The organisation has identified through its computer software system that a small proportion of the enrolees (less than 1%) are responsible for up to 25% of medical costs. The organisation therefore operates intensive case management delivered via telephone by nurses to these patients. The case management service provides early identification and support for the patients.

Touchpoint Health Plan (Wisconsin)

This organisation is owned by two 'for-profit' companies, and provides a wide range of services underpinned by an ethos of quality improvement and a mission to improve health across communities. The organisation has extended its chronic disease management activities with incentives for physicians to achieve quality levels and deliver appropriate care. The organisation does not stratify or identify patients at risk but it does employ case managers who work closely with primary care and specialist clinicians who work with poorly controlled patients.

Anthem Blue Cross and Blue Shield (Connecticut)

Anthem is an organisation formed in 1997 from a number of earlier organisations, and it became a for-profit organisation in 2001. It provides a mix of tightly- and loosely control managed care processes. The organisation case manages catastrophic care for enrolees and case manages the top 1% of patients with most complex medical needs. These complex patients are identified by the software system, which collates information on claims and other data. The organisation also offer programmes for specific chronic diseases (diabetes, asthma, cardio vascular disease) including self-care and regular reviews with bonuses for clinicians who achieve clinical targets.

UnitedHealth Europe Evercare

The Evercare programme began as a small local government project in 1987 and is now a national programme, which provides a model of proactive case management to 71,000 people within nursing homes and the community. The programmes aimed specifically at case management are based on stratification of patients and levels of intervention, particularly those with complex needs, that is the upper level of the Kaiser processes. The advanced primary nurses role is clearly defined by Evercare and evaluated positively. The processes used within the case management are outlined as care orchestration, communication, acting as a champion or advocate, showing high-level clinical skills and acting as a coach. These skills are seen as fundamental to managing these complex patients, enabling care to be managed across the care pathway with effective communication. Once identified, high-risk patients are assessed and their care is then planned using anticipatory processes.

Amsterdam HealthCare System (the Netherlands) [5]

The health system within the Netherlands was funded initially through insurance with three compartments: first compartment includes uninsured and unpayable risks, for example health care for the chronically sick and the elderly; second compartment includes curative care (general practice and hospital care), which is dual funded; and the third compartment includes supplementary care (requiring voluntary insurance). Since the reform of health insurance in 2006 all residents are insured for the standard package of care through a basic national insurance (Volksverzekering), which is means tested and taken from gross income. In addition, a sickness fund (Zeikenfonds), which is also a means tested payment, is also paid on yearly income. The latter provided general practice and consultant care including investigations and other supportive care but there may be some additional charges for specific medication. There are choice elements that are managed through private insurance. There has in recent years been a push within the Dutch health system to reduce institutionalisation, improve patient empowerment, increase ambulatory care, develop the processes of integration and increase competition and market forces. Many of the providers are not-for-profit organisations with, where possible, an integrated and partnership (networks) approach to care delivery. The Dutch healthcare system recognises the increasing burden of chronic diseases and the increasing cost of health care. In 2004 60 million Euros (12.8% of gross domestic product [GDP]) were spent on health care in the Netherlands. Life expectancy is expected to rise from 75.5 to 78 years in men and from 80.6 to 81.7 years in women, and as in all other countries the prevalence of chronic disease is also expected to increase [6].

Although the provision of care is similar to the UK system, with general practice as the gatekeeper to all care, it is in some ways different, with the use of a personal budget system, which increases flexibility of service provision and enables personalised care planning. The key themes for the Dutch healthcare system are improving public health, reducing the prevalence of long-term conditions and improving outcomes for those with long-term conditions; these themes are similar to those within the NHS. Within the Dutch systems all patients are listed with a general practice, similar to the United Kingdom system, and the models of care delivery in primary care are focused on continuity, co-ordination and comprehensive services. There are in the healthcare system providers who deliver the management of long-term conditions, providing full service from diagnostics to regular review, including call and recall, and management, including all required screening. The information from this system is reported immediately into the general practice clinical systems and deviations from expected goals for care can then be managed as appropriate. The system does not at this time have case management models as delivered with the US system but it does provide care intervention for chronic disease in primary care or via specialist providers and ambulatory and rehabilitative services aimed at promoting and enabling independence for patients with chronic disease and disability.

Outcome intervention model (New Zealand)

In the New Zealand model, the government is using an outcomes intervention process, which sets four final outcomes (better health, reduced inequalities, better participation and independence, and trust and security) and then outlines the levels of interventions needed to deliver the outcomes. Supporting this process a number of models of care are also being trialled, many of which contain elements of the chronic care model. The models with co-ordinated care from a multidisciplinary team have proved to be most effective.

National model of chronic disease prevention and control (Australia)

Australia has had a clearly defined public health framework since 2001 that has emphasised on prevention and promotion. The Australian model of care for chronic diseases focuses on delivery along the continuum of disease. It starts from primary prevention in the healthy population through to secondary prevention and early detection in the at-risk population, and finally, to disease management for established disease, and management and tertiary prevention for those with complex chronic disease. All areas of intervention are underpinned by health promotion, which is aimed at disease prevention as (rather than in) the patient moves along the disease continuum. There are differing strategies across some of the regions but all aim to improve access, reduce health inequalities and improve outcomes for patients with chronic conditions through self-care, continuity and quality of care provision.

Guided Care (United States)

Guided Care is a model similar to the community matron role in the England. This model delivers comprehensive assessment and care planning, care co-ordination, best practice for chronic diseases, self-care, healthy lifestyles advice and information and support for families and carers for older people with multiple conditions through Guided Care Nurses working in partnership with primary care physicians. The outcomes for this model – reduced resource use and improved quality of life – are similar to those of other models.

PACE (United States)

The Program of All-Inclusive Care for the Elderly (PACE) is a care model that aims to reduce use of hospital and nursing home care in the elderly. The model identifies patients using day centres and through an integrated approach enables care to be provided in a way that ensures continuity and communication.

Veterans Affairs (Unites States)

Veterans Affairs health organisation provides care for a large part of the ex-service personnel in the United States. It has an expanded model of chronic disease care with additional processes for health promotion and prevention. The provider organisation claims that the care model provides improved quality of care, reduced resource use and improved clinical outcomes.

Improving Chronic Illness Care (Seattle) [7]

This process is not a service delivery model as such but is an assessment of effectiveness for both design and efficacy of provision. The methodology was developed to complete a service review of a well-established diabetes service within the United States. It was further developed to provide a process for assessment of current levels of care within service. This methodology utilises the components of the chronic care model (used by many, if not all, of the managed care providers) and allows the organisations to evaluate outcomes and understand areas for improvement. The process has been utilised effectively by the Institute for Healthcare Improvement in the United States to guide organisations on how to improve service quality.

Expanded Chronic Care Model (Canada)

In Canada, policymakers adapted the chronic care model that focussed on clinic-orientated systems to include prevention and health promotion activities. The processes included in this model allow population health promotion to be linked to social determinants of health and enhanced participation in communities. This adaptation has allowed the delivery of population-based care alongside individualised care.

Pfizer (United States)

The Pfizer model targets care to the highest risk patients and supplements existing service users' telephone contacts to monitor and refer those patients. The strategies used are identification of those at risk, case finding, patient education, proactive management of patients, dedicated telephone support from nurses and telephone case management software (information technology), which included national and local guidelines.

Green Ribbon Health: Medicare in health support (Florida) [8]

This programme of care for older people with multiple chronic conditions such as diabetes and congestive health failure is delivered within the state of Florida in the United States [8]. The programme targets customised interventions based on health need. Users are assessed and provided with an individualised programme of care and support; this is based on risk stratification. The model is delivered using a patient engagement model through telephone support and community-based multidisciplinary teams. The levels of intervention are designed based on need and risk and these interventions aim to improve functionality. This model utilises decision support software via an IT platform. The model has provided improvements in patient outcomes, quality and patient safety.

What do these models provide?

It is clear from this short review that all the organisations are aiming to provide similar improvements in cost containment, care quality and outcomes. Each organisation appears to be aiming towards integration of prevention and treatment and attempting to define needs based on the total population. Fundamental to the delivery of all the care models is the presence of high-quality clinical leadership, evidence-based practice/care and development and maintenance of disease registers. The importance of the relationship between professionals and excellent communications is also clearly outlined, as is the importance of public reporting of outcomes. Another process that does appear in all models to provide improvements in care is the use of incentives.

Models in use in England

PCTs in the NHS have a significant advantage on the US healthcare organisations in improving the management of long-term conditions because of the number of national strategies, implementation programmes and National Service Frameworks (NSFs). The January 2005 publication 'Supporting people with long term conditions' by the DH outlines the government's plans to support people with long-term conditions live healthy lives and presents an NHS and social care model based on the good practice within the United Kingdom and abroad. This document outlines the challenge and opportunities for the NHS in relation to chronic disease management. The key facets of the NHS model are as follows:

- A systematic approach that links health, social care, patients and carers;
- Identify everyone with a long-term condition;
- Stratify people so that they can receive care according to their needs;
- Focus on frequent users of secondary care services;

- Use community matrons to provide case management;
- Develop ways to identify people who may become very high intensity users;
- Establish multidisciplinary teams in primary care supported by specialist advice;
- Develop local ways to support self-care;
- Expand the Expert Patient Programme and other self-management programmes;
- Use tools and techniques already available to make an impact.

The model also defines the infrastructure (community resources, decision support tools and clinical information and health and social care environment) required, the delivery system (case management, disease management, supported self-care and better health promotion) and better outcomes (empowered and informed patients, prepared and proactive health and social care teams). The areas in which the NHS is seen as less able than the US systems to support improvements in care of long-term conditions are lower levels of customer focus, less use of incentives, particularly for innovation, and continued central pressure to deliver on targets.

The use of Evercare within England was predicated on a process that aligns the model with pathways and processes included in NSFs. The initial reviews highlighted a number of areas in which the Evercare model would deliver specific outcomes required with particularly the NSF for Older People [9]. The standards reviewed for delivery were as follows:

- Standard 2: person-centred care;
- Standard 3: intermediate care;
- Standard 4: general hospital care;
- Standard 7: mental health in older people;
- Standard 8: the promotion of active life in older age.

The NHS while developing its pilots for Evercare clearly reviewed the core principles the model espouses to ensure these were deliverable within NHS and social care structures, and if not, then what new/additional infrastructure would be required. Prior to implementation, the NHS also completed a review on alignment of the NHS Plan with the key policy drivers [9]. This provided an overview of how implementation of this model of care would deliver a number of key initiatives within the plan, including spearheading clinical innovation in care, improving use of scarce resources and focusing on people's health. A pathway for service implementation was already clearly outlined by United HealthCare and mapping this locally against implementation to ensure alignment clearly affected the success of implementation. This process of alignment provided Evercare and the NHS with some clear evidence on the need for redesign of the programme to enable effective outcomes. The specific areas identified for local flavour were role development and re-engineering, development of data processes to identify appropriate patients and re-engineering for some interventions to improve capacity to manage high-risk older patients.

Care management in social care

Since the implementation of the Community Care Act in 1990 care management has been in place across local authorities in England. The processes that enable the delivery of care management in social care are similar to those outlined in case management models. These processes are well established in social care and are focused on assessment of need, planning and implementation of care based on the need, with monitoring of success and review. The processes for care management were identified from earlier reviews of care for frail elderly people with multiple disabilities. The main deliverers of care management have been qualified social workers, but full implementation has not been achieved for a number of reasons. Specific skills and training [10] for care management roles were developed and delivered in the 1990s and then added to social work training.

Case management models in the NHS

The DH published 'Supporting people with long term conditions' in January 2005 [11], which outlined a health and social care model that enabled organisations to take a structured and systematic approach to managing people with long-term conditions. The model outlines processes that support delivery divided into three areas: infrastructure, delivery systems and outcomes. Infrastructure such as community resources, clinical information systems including decision support tools and integrated care environment are seen as supporting the delivery systems. The delivery systems at the three levels across the disease process supported self-care, disease management and case management and thus delivered the improved patient outcomes of empowered and informed patients alongside proactive health and social care teams. These levels of intervention will enable targeting of care through appropriate levels of skills and competence. At each of these levels of care, intervention is based on the degree of need, and it is delivered by staff with the appropriate knowledge and skills. The levels of care needed are identified as progressively increasing from supported self-care, through disease-specific management to case management. The development of services based on these models of care is underpinned by the identification of the population, redesign of care processes and delivery and the effective measurement of outcomes and feedback on care. An understanding of the population within a local health economy enables the commissioning of appropriate service for all levels of need, from diagnosis and self-care through to palliative care.

   The DH developed a framework for implementation of Evercare models with 10 PCTs through an assessment of capacity and readiness and development of implementation pilots. The results from pilots across the NHS were fairly successful and the National Primary Care Trust development programme (natpact.nhs.uk) has produced on their website some feedbacks from the Evercare project sites. The feedbacks are divided into the following five areas:

- Changing roles
- Patient focus
- Data
- Relationships
- Miscellaneous

In each of these areas, clearly positive progress and responses are reported. In relation to role changes, it is clear that these pilots saw this as an excellent opportunity to move from medical to preventative models of care, to expand nursing and other roles and as a catalyst for service modernisation. In relation to patient focus, the positives are increasing focus on people and their carers and movement of care closer to the community and patients. A number of positive factors with regard to relationships are also outlined, including strengthening connections with social care and closer cooperation between general practitioners and nurses and acute and primary care. Despite the positive feedback there were a number of major challenges including funding, time and capacity to develop skills in advanced nursing roles, lack of data in relation to both evidence of impact and what data to collect. Other key issues were the timescales pilots were completed in and the work required to gain the hearts and minds of the general practitioners and other medical staff.

Since the development of pilots of case management across the NHS, all organisations have been developing their own models of chronic disease management. All PCTs have been charged with the development of strategies to implement models of care through commissioning and service redesign to achieve the expected improvements in care. Many PCTs have published long-term conditions strategies and plans that outline how appropriate models of care will be implemented by their local providers. All these plans and strategies outline the size of the problem in their local area and the impact on the health of the population. Most models in use within the plans and strategies are based to a greater or lesser degree on the Pfizer levels of care and Evercare processes, but many organisations have localised this to ensure effective implementation based on local needs.

During the pilot programme, UnitedHealth Care identified that NHS organisations were data rich but information poor [12]. All organisation have therefore spent time focusing on how to improve this situation through improved information technology systems. Organisations within the Birmingham and Black Country Strategic Health Authority (SHA) have developed a web-enabled case management database that allows information input from general practice and acute providers, and case managers could access this information via a web address. This data system allows quality data storage and automated reporting [13]. This functionality has allowed the organisations involved to measure and report improvements in many areas relating to long-term conditions.

Central Manchester PCT has developed a team approach to active case management of chronic disease [14]. The model is based on a broad multidisciplinary team, which is formed from a local area team of case managers and assistant practitioners linked to a virtual team including pharmacists, district nurses, allied health professionals and intermediate care and mental health staff. The roles of lead case manager and case manager are planned to allow the lead case manager to predict and manage the patients with highly complex needs and the case manager to manage the patients with medium to low complexity. This model of care delivers active case management for patients at levels 2 and 3 of the Pfizer model of care and is supported by improved access to diagnostics and rehabilitation services. This model clearly outlines the way in which caseloads will be identified and managed, and based on the findings from the Evercare pilot, this is an important process to ensure effective outcomes.

Cheshire and Merseyside SHA completed a review of all local PCTs' state of readiness for implementation of case management programmes; it was published in January 2005. This review identified that many of the organisations had made progress in their developments but most were struggling with full implementation owing to lack of robust data to allow the identification of high-risk patients and caseloads. The organisations involved in this review had embraced the changes required to deliver the new models of care and most had started developing their programmes of care, but in most cases the ability to report outcomes through their data systems was proving problematic.

The organisations within Cheshire and Merseyside were also clear that case management should not be seen as a panacea for all ills and that a focus on the top 3% of patients (the high-intensity users) may be successful for these patients but did not provide any improvements for those in the lower levels, who without substantial improvements in care will eventually join the ranks of high intensity users. The organisations within Cheshire and Merseyside have also worked together to develop an SHA-wide job description for a nurse case manager (community matron) and a generic case manager (nurse and allied health professional), which enabled some consistency of approach across the organisations. The organisations worked in collaboration with all local universities to develop a local education programme, which was delivered via all the local higher education institutions. The development of this programme based on the educational outcomes set within the national competencies at master's level provides all students with a post-graduate diploma in long-term conditions; case managers in all organisations were encouraged to attend this programme.

The staff involved within the three PCTs in Bristol and South Gloucester as part of the Evercare pilot in 2004, and who implemented case management, have identified the core principles that proved most effective for them. These are reported as treatment focused on the individual person, which preserves independence, function and quality of life and care delivered in the least invasive manner in the least intensive setting as possible. These core principles link well with all of the policy drivers for health and social care. The model was delivered through advanced nurse practitioners who were linked to appropriate primary care practitioners and specialist teams. The success of this part of the pilot was monitored through feedback from patients, carers, families and staff involved in the service, which delivered some positive outcomes in terms of patient and carer satisfaction. Case management had a positive effect on medication usage and concordance, and lengths of stay and emergency admissions were reduced. These findings were then utilised to inform commissioning decisions for the future [15].

Luton PCT has implemented case management led by community matrons. The caseload for these staff was identified via the Patients at Risk of Re-hospitalisation (PARR) tool and an agreed local threshold for repeated admission to hospital. The outcomes of the system delivered a net saving on £81,000 per community matron from reduced inpatient admissions, a reduction in average length of stay from 14 days to 6 days and high levels of improved outcomes and patient satisfaction. More than 80% of patients felt more able to cope with their condition and felt that their health care was better organised, also 90% felt they had a better understanding of their condition [16].

It is understood that people with long-term conditions with a range of complex needs will require care from many different professionals, and bringing together of multidisciplinary teams is seen as crucial to providing a seamless co-ordinated approach to care. The implementation of these teams avoids fragmentation of care and reduces duplication of effort for patients and staff. Many organisations across the NHS have developed and implemented these teams with evidence of excellent outcomes owing to better understanding of roles and functions, implementation of single assessment process and joint records, flexible referral processes, encouragement of innovation and shared ownership of care, and despite some tensions between universal access to health and eligibility to social care, preventative care has been delivered.

The implementation of individual budgets and direct payments in health is currently under debate but these budget processes have been available in social care for sometime. Direct payments uptake in social care has been not as effective in some areas as expected, but where it has been utilised the impact on choice and independence is highly valued by the clients. Barnsley PCT and Adult Social Service have developed a vision for adult health, independence and well-being in their strategy 'Every Adult Matters', which allows the provision of care and support for individuals based on self-assessment, self-management and choice through individual budgets [16].

Numerous other organisations have developed their case management models, producing long-term condition strategies and teams including community matrons and other case management roles. All the models clearly focus, in the first instance, on identifying appropriate services and supports for patients who are high users of services. Implementation appears to be most successful in those areas where planning for the process is robust and has included processes for engagement across health and social care, including acute and primary care medics. Other key impacts on success have been clear role definition, good infrastructure including 24-hr access to community nursing and robust intermediate care services, multidisciplinary team working and good social care links/integration.

In Cornwall and the Isles of Scilly, first-quarter EPIC (Elderly Care Project in Cornwall) report [17] clearly outlines the process through which the service has been developed and the impact the service has had on specific patients. Even at this early stage it is clear that outcomes for patients are positive with a number of prevented admissions and much improved patient satisfaction. Greater Manchester PCT reported to their board on their plans for the implementation of active case management based on the chronic disease management models and care pyramid. The organisation had clearly reviewed the processes it will need to implement a locally responsive service for proactive case management. A number of SHAs produced frameworks and strategies for long-term conditions. Essex published [18] a framework and service directory that while proffering advice did not specify a service model for PCTs to implement. It did require each organisation to produce an implementation plan, including a workforce development plan for roll out.

Warrington PCT has developed for clients with learning disabilities, who are likely to be at a higher risk of long-term health problems, a service based on an anticipatory care calendar. The programme utilises care management skills to proactively plan and deliver care to this client group. The planning enables appropriate screening and general health reviews to be completed effectively and in a planned way, which, in turn, enables improvements in care for this difficult to manage client group.

Team Haringey is delivering a model of care in partnership with Pfizer [19]. The project was developed as part of a transformational change programme and was completed as part of a wider project to reform local services for patients with long-term conditions. The programme utilises a decision support package and involves initial assessment of patients by telephone, which was followed up with interventions provided via case manager practitioners (nurses).

East Lincolnshire PCT developed and delivered a model of case management for patients with chronic obstructive airways disease [20]. The model enables management across the pathway of care. The model aims to improve care in a high-priority area of the PCT. In this model, a specialist team has been integrated with generalist teams to enable holistic care delivery. The model enables quality services that are safe and effective. The programme was able to report a 23% reduction in chronic obestructive pulmonary disease (COPD) admissions and enabled improved management of acute exacerbations within the community. It is hoped that this service will deliver a 50% reduction in hospital admissions.

Joint NHS and social care

A number of organisations have developed integration models of care delivery for adults or children. Knowsley PCT, in partnership with Knowsley Metropolitan Borough Council that had already integrated many of their key roles and functions, produced a joint long-term conditions strategy in October 2005 [21]. It clearly outlined their intentions regarding how they would commission service delivery based on the chronic care model. This strategy outlines the plans for service delivery across all levels of the care pyramid, from prevention to case management.

The development of joint/integrated care services for patients with long-term and chronic conditions is obviously a major step forward and the DH has been supporting a number of pilots in organisations around the United Kingdom [22]. These local authorities and PCTs have already commenced a process of integration to enable a more logical approach to service delivery, reducing transfers and hand offs and of course sharing responsibility for ensuring ongoing independence. There is evidence that targeting support for these individuals can deliver improved cost effectiveness of care and improve health outcomes and independence. The targeted support is described as follows:

- Putting the individuals' needs at the centre of service provision by promoting long-term independence, improving quality of life, ensuring clinical and cost effectiveness and addressing equality and diversity issues;
- Supporting the user with improved co-ordination of care (collaboration across health, social care and housing);
- Using assistive technologies.

The requirement in this model is for all systems to be integrated, that is joint needs assessment, commissioning and planning, performance management and delivery by joint teams, supported by integrated information technology and records. It is expected that these integrated services will deliver care focused on people rather than place of care, empowerment of patients, robust management of risk and sustainable development.

A number of other approaches to case management have also been implemented. In Croydon PCT [23], two virtual wards of 100 patients have been developed. This service is based within primary care and is linked directly to general practices but is organised like a hospital ward; its structure and support includes a ward clerk type post as central link to communicate across the professionals and carers who are delivering care to the patients. Norfolk has taken an approach based on prevention rather than cure. In their approach patients who are at risk of becoming high-intensity users are targeted using telephone coaching and support to improve their abilities to self-manage. The approach in Norfolk is delivered via the Norfolk Health Line, which provides patients with the ability and confidence to share the decision making relating for their care. The model aims to provide direct advice available by telephone to facilitate self-care and knowledge of their disease.

Intensive case management model in Greater Peterborough Primary Care Trust Partnership delivered targeted interventions for patients who fitted a discrete set of criteria: aged over 75 years, three or more admissions in last six months, three or more conditions and five or more medications. The programme delivered intensive case management (health care) and care management (social care) in partnership across health and social care. The model was successful in reducing emergency admissions.

Data for case management

The identification of very high intensity users for proactive case management has, as outlined earlier, proved slightly difficult and many case management services have struggled to do so effectively. Although all patients with a long-term condition are appropriate for some form of proactive case management based on the long-term conditions models of care outlined earlier, it is clear that those patients who are the highest users of health and social care services are the focus for DH policy as it is only through reduction of emergency admissions in this group that the Public Service Agreement (PSA) targets will be achieved.

The NHS has through a project commissioned by the DH from the King's Fund and its collaborators [24] developed a predictive risk algorithm using a broad range of data to identify appropriate patients. The ongoing attempts to identify patients have led to the development of a tool to predict the patients who will require emergency care, and the tool appears to do this effectively. The tool developed identifies patients across a continuum of risk in line with the long-term conditions pyramid and this information can then be utilised to target interventions that are appropriate to the need. The project was developed based on the information from two PCTs with 560,000 patients, which included Hospital Episode Statistics (HES) data and inpatient (IP), outpatient (OP), accident and emergency (A&E) and general practice (GP) electronic records. This tool appears to have a high degree of accuracy in relation to identification of patients at risk of future emergency admission but who have not previously been admitted. Early versions of the tool appeared to predict those at risk of readmission. The model indicates that if organisations were to provide robust interventions for 250 high-risk patents at a cost of approximately £500.00 per patient, there would be a potential saving of £92,920.00 on reduced hospitals admissions. Some organisations across the NHS have utilised a variety of models of prediction to identify patients for case management caseloads, including supplementing predictive data models with supporting knowledge of patients via professionals who are currently involved in their care.

Evaluation

All the models outlined aim to deliver improvements in patient outcomes, including a reduction in acute care usage, and all are based on some form of identification of high-risk patients and co-ordination of care. The models across the different countries are broadly similar in aim though slightly different in delivery in line with the healthcare system in which they are being delivered. The most effective case management models appear to be those that are appropriately planned, linked to other services and supported by clinicians. It is also clear from this discussion that there are a number of possible models that can be used. These models of care management can and are very effective, but they are not a panacea. The implementation of care models must reflect the needs of specific populations, they must be flexible and, to be fully effective, they must be focused on an appropriately identified caseload. In all the evaluations of case management models, a key to success has been the ability to identify the appropriate patient caseload, which has proved difficult in many areas. Even in the United Healthcare (Evercare) pilot areas, it is clear that information needed to identify these patients was a difficult to find, as the NHS was seen to have poor information systems. Within the NHS a number of information systems have been developed to identify appropriate patients and although these are being used across organisations and are subject to ongoing review, none of them are seen as fully successful in identifying appropriate patients. In the most effective programmes, a mix of IT-based and clinically influenced patient identification system are being utilised. The development improved information systems in PCTs to support commissioning and of course the practice based commissioning (PBC) consortia would potentially offer an opportunity to identify an appropriate patient caseload.

Within the evaluations other keys to success are the competence of the practitioners, the presence of excellent supportive functions (social care, diagnostics), support and links to primary care, medical support to practitioners and access to multidisciplinary teams. The competence of practitioners enables early identification of changes in condition, recognition of risks and their management, which will ensure the safety of patients. The ability of practitioners involved to deliver advanced clinical skills in examination and diagnostics is important to ensure that patients are appropriately and safely managed.

If practitioners are to be effective, they must be able to develop good working relationships across health and social care at all levels as they need to develop and maintain the confidence of, particularly, medical colleagues to ensure trust in their assessments and decision making. The level of confidence practitioners have in their knowledge base will affect their ability to communicate with medical colleagues in acute and primary care and will also affect the confidence of patients and carers. The support to case management practitioners by medical colleagues either during education and training or in the ongoing delivery of care to support competency review is fundamental as it provides a high level of credibility.

In the development of case management, organisations need to ensure that practitioners can access appropriate diagnostics, as often a reason for admission can be lack of access to diagnostics. The same is true for access to intermediate care or step up beds for planned admission to manage care problems that are medically stable and do not require acute care. It also appears to be very important that during the development of the model of care appropriate stakeholders are included in the discussions and planning. Clinical engagement is therefore fundamental as without this the support and credibility will not be in place.

Patient- and carer-reported outcomes in relation to case management are very positive. Patients feel that having a practitioner with whom they can develop a relationship and who they can trust to provide the communication between acute and other care provider are seen as being very effective. The co-ordination role between care providers and families or personal carers is also seen as a highly effective function. In general term, patients report feeling more confident in their care, having a better understanding of and compliance with medication and feeling better supported. In balance of the patient views, it is understood that any service that provides specific focused care to a patient will impact positively as the positive feedback from the patient may be linked to this.

The evaluations completed and reported did not necessarily deliver the level of acute admission savings expected in all areas. But they did provide evidence of improved outcomes for patients:

- Reduced medication-related issues;
- Reduced length of stay following admission;
- Increased planned admissions;
- Reduced general practitioners' home visits and out of hours call outs;
- Increased patient confidence in management of care and self-management;
- Increased carer support.

Although this evaluation did not prove delivery on all expectations, it did provide evidence of improved outcomes for both patients and carers. As mentioned earlier in this discussion, it is important that plans for management of chronic conditions deal with delivery of care across all the levels of need not just the top of the pyramid of care. The development of strategic commissioning plans within PCTs will probably include the services at all levels of the chronic disease model, including prevention and the promotion of screening, early diagnosis and self-care/behavioural change. Ongoing evaluation of all service provisions is a requirement of new commissioning processes and this must be a requirement for all care management-based services to ensure continued effectiveness and development of improved models of care.

Conclusion

The development of models of case management is at the heart of the modernisation of the NHS and it is clear that case management models offer a huge opportunity to improve outcomes for patients. Models of case management have been proved to be effective internationally and partially effective within the NHS. As case management services develop and the NHS continues on its progress towards modernisation, case management will probably be one of the fundamental tools in improving patient outcomes and access to services. The delivery of high-quality care to patients with long-term conditions does not have one service model answer, there needs to be a clear assessment of needs and modelling of services must be based on those needs.

References

1. Warner J, Lewis R and Gillam S (2001). *US Managed Care and PCTs: Lessons from a Small Island to a Lost Continent*. King's Fund. http://www.kingsfund.org.uk/applications/site_search/?term=Lessons+from+a+small+island&searchreferer_id=2&submit.x=19&submit.y=16 (accessed on October 2009).
2. Dixon J, Lewis R, Rosen R, Finlayson B and Gray D (2004). *Managing Chronic Disease: What We can Learn from the US Experience*. King's Fund. http://www.kingsfund.org.uk/research/publications/managing_chronic.html (accessed on October 2009).
3. Harding M (2005). *The Alaskan Medical Service: Report of a Visit*. Association of Greater Manchester Primary Care Trusts. (www.greatermanchester.nhs.uk)
4. Department of Health (September 2005). *Kaiser Permanente Report on the Visit to San Francisco Cheshire & Merseyside Strategic Health Authority*.
5. van den Bos GAM (2005). *Dutch Healthcare System and Arrangements for Managing Long Term Conditions: Information for Study Tour*. Academic Medical Centre of Amsterdam. (www.man.ac.uk)
6. UnitedHealth Europe (2006). *Assessment of Evercare Programme in England 2003–2004*. http://www.dh.gov.uk/prod_consum_dh/groups/dh_digitalassets/@dh/@en/documents/digitalasset/dh_4114224.pdf (accessed on October 2009).
7. Institute for Healthcare Improvement (2004). *Improving Chronic Illness Care: A National Programme of Robert Wood Johnson Foundation, USA*. http://www.ihi.org/IHI/Topics/ChronicConditions/Asthma/Resources/ImprovingChronicIllnessCare.htm (accessed on October 2009).
8. Lord J.T. King's Fund (2007). *Green Ribbon Health Improving Care for High Costs Patients with Complex Chronic Conditions*. http://www.kingsfund.org.uk/applications/site_search/?term=Green+ribbon+health&searchreferer_id=10204&submit.x=41&submit.y=13 (accessed on October 2009).
9. Evercare United Healthcare Group (2003). *Adapting the Evercare Programme for the National Health Service*. http://www.dh.gov.uk/prod_consum_dh/groups/dh_digitalassets/@dh/@en/documents/digitalasset/dh_4114224.pdf
10. Department of Health, Social Services Inspectorate (1991). *Care Management and Assessment: Practitioners Guide*. HMSO London.
11. Department of Health (2005). *Supporting People with Long Term Conditions: An NHS and Social Model to Support Local Innovation and Integration*. http://www.dh.gov.uk/prod_consum_dh/groups/dh_digitalassets/@dh/@en/documents/digitalasset/dh_4122574.pdf (accessed on October 2009).
12. UnitedHealth Europe (February 2005). *Assessment of the Evercare Programme in England 2003 to 2004*. http://www.dh.gov.uk/prod_consum_dh/groups/dh_digitalassets/@dh/@en/documents/digitalasset/dh_4114224.pdf
13. Dudley Beacon and Castle Primary Care Trust (2006). *Web Enabled Community Case Management Database*. (www.dudley.nhs.uk)
14. Central Manchester Primary Care Trust (2005). *Development of Teams for Active Case Management of Chronic Disease*. Board presentation. (www.centralmanchester.nhs.uk)
15. *The Bristol and South Gloucestershire Evercare Programme: Presentation of Outcomes*, November 2004. (www.bristol.nhs.uk)
16. Department of Health (2008). *Raising the Profile of Long Term Conditions Care: A Compendium of Information*. http://www.dh.gov.uk/prod_consum_dh/groups/dh_digitalassets/documents/digitalasset/dh_082067.pdf (accessed on October 2009).
17. Cornwall and Isles of Scilly Health & Social Care Community (2004). *Eldercare Project in Cornwall: First Quarter Evaluation*. (www.cornwall.nhs.uk)

18. Essex Strategic Health Authority (December 2004). *Strategic Framework for Case Management of Long Term Conditions*. http://www.dhsspsni.gov.uk/case_management.pdf

19. Harrington S (2007). *TeamHealth: Long-Term Conditions Partnership Pilot between Harringey Teaching PCT and Pfizer*. King's Fund. http://www.kingsfund.org.uk/applications/site_search/?term=TeamHealth&oldterm=Pfizer&old_term=Pfizer&old_instance_id=181636&submit.x=30&submit.y=13

20. O'Kelly N (2006). *Managing Patients Across the Care Pathway: East Lincolnshire Chronic Obstructive Pulmonary Disease Service*. King's Fund. http://www.kingsfund.org.uk/applications/site_search/?term=Managing+across+a+care+pathway&searchreferer_id=0&searchreferer_url=%2Fapplications%2Fsite_search%2Findex.rm&submit.x=39&submit.y=9 (accessed on October 2009).

21. Knowsley Primary Care Trust (2005) *Integrating to Improve Services: Knowsley Long Term Conditions Strategy 2005–2008*. Commissioning Group. (www.knowsley.nhs.uk)

22. Department of Health (December 2006). Whole Systems Long Term Conditions Demonstrators. http://www.dh.gov.uk/en/Healthcare/Longtermconditions/wholesystemdemonstrators/index.htm (accessed on October 2009).

23. Lepper J (February 2007). Creating virtual wards in the community. *Independent Nurse*. 19th February 2007 Vol 23 page 56–58.

24. Health Dialog, King's Fund and New York University Center for Health and Public Services (2006). *Combined Predictive Model: Executive Summary of Interim Results*. http://www.kingsfund.org.uk/applications/site_search/?term=Combined+Model+Executive+summary+of+interim+results&oldterm=Health+dialog&old_term=Health+dialog&old_instance_id=180491&submit.x=19&submit.y=8 (accessed on October 2009).

Chapter 3
Competencies for Managing Long-Term Conditions

Introduction

All professional regulators clearly outline the knowledge skills and expertise they expect the members of the profession to have on entry into the profession. These skills and expertise form the educational outcomes that are then developed to underpin training. These processes provide the bedrock on which the professionals are then further developed to be 'fit for purpose', that is to enable to develop the increasingly complex skills required by the care delivery models. However, the skills professionals develop within basic training are in the main baseline and generalist in approach, and do not always provide the advanced or specific skills required for specialist areas or advance level interventions. It is well recognised that timely and appropriate intervention from an appropriately skilled workforce can and will ensure effective care, quality and safety and of course improved outcomes and patient satisfaction.

The dictionary definition of competent is 'adequate, sufficiently able, properly qualified', it is therefore clear that being competent is fundamental for a professional to deliver care.

The World Health Organisation [1] defines competence as follows:

> Competence requires knowledge, appropriate attitudes and observable mechanical or intellectual skills which together account for the ability to deliver a professional service.

Eraut [2] defines competence as socially defined or individually situated competence. He suggests that socially defined competence is that which is applied at any stage of the career and is the expectation to perform at an expected standard. Whereas individually situated competency relates to what he describes as 'criterion-referenced effective and superior performance'.

Competence therefore could be seen as follows:

- Knowledge and understanding;
- Skills (cognitive/technical/psychomotor/interpersonal);
- Personal attributes.

The Royal College of Nursing (RCN) [3] clearly outlines a view of competency as being evidence that a nurse possesses the skills and abilities required to work in a safe and effective professional way that is in line with the law. The RCN utilises in its definitions of competence the guidance from the Department of Health (DH) [4] in relation to the levels of nursing practice and is clear that evidence is required of competency achievement and maintenance.

Therefore, to provide safe and effective care, the staff delivering care must hold appropriate levels of knowledge, skills, expertise and personal attributes that enable them to be competent. Within the care environments and particularly in the National Health Service (NHS), the issue of ensuring staff are employed with appropriate abilities for their roles and functions, and that they continue to maintain these, is seen as essential for the delivery of effective care. All roles within the NHS are designed with job descriptions and person specifications and are expected to be underpinned by a process known as the Knowledge and Skills Framework (KSF) [5].

The KSF outlines in six main domains and a number of specific domains the skills and knowledge required within a job role. The KSF is classified into a foundation outline (skills and knowledge expected in a new post holder) and a full outline (skills and knowledge expected in a professional fully functioning within the post). Unfortunately, the KSF does not provide any formal basis against which an educational programme or learning outcomes can be developed. However, the set of competencies outlined for a role would provide sufficient information and guidance to allow the development of 'learning outcomes' on which programmes for educational training or ongoing development can be prepared. The need to ensure competencies are defined and met is clearly recognised and many authors and investigations into care failures in the NHS have articulated this need [5–7].

Development of the competency framework

All educational programmes within the professions are now developed from the standards of practice and competencies outlined and agreed by the appropriate professional regulators. The NHS has developed a structured set of competencies as part of an educational framework [8] for staff working with patients with long-term conditions. The educational framework clearly defines the competencies that are required by the staff to support patients with these conditions. The framework 'Caring for people with long-term conditions: an education framework for community matrons and case managers' was published in 2006 [9] and provided an outline of the case management competencies and an educational framework to facilitate the development and maintenance of these competencies. The NHS Modernisation Agency and Skills for Health [10] had in 2005 outlined the knowledge and skills for professionals responsible for the care of people with long-term conditions, and this work was utilised to underpin the development of the educational framework. A broad range of clinicians, educationalists, patient representatives, senior managers and policymakers were involved in the development of the framework. The educational framework is aimed at enabling competency development in all staff working with patients with long-term conditions. In this framework, staff are outlined as case managers, who could be a nurse, social worker or allied health professional or a community matron, who is seen as a nursing role with the advanced practice requirements set by the Nursing Midwifery Council [10]. All roles are expected to function within an appropriate professional regulatory framework. The competency framework for case management fits with the ongoing development of competencies across the workforce, which is being supported through the National Workforce Projects and Skills for Health.

The National Workforce Projects have themselves released a framework of competencies for workforce planners within the NHS to assist in its strategic workforce planning [11].

The competency framework for case management describes competencies within nine domains, including an Advanced Clinical Nursing Practice domain, relating to community matron-type roles, and eight domains for case managers who do not provide these advanced nursing interventions. The domains within the framework are outlined in Table 3.1 (based on information in Ref. [9]) Within each domain there are further explanations for each subset within the specific competence.

The competency framework can and has in many organisations been used to recruit appropriately skilled staff. The tools can also be used in the assessment of the existing staffs' levels of knowledge and skills, providing an analysis of the educational and training needs. The competencies are also seen as a tool with which ongoing assessment of performance can be enabled; workforce needs can be identified and planned for through commissioning of education to re-skill or up-skill staff.

The framework has also been useful for higher educational institutions in the development of educational programmes for training staff or providers of care so that they are fully capable of delivering care and are seen as 'fit for purpose'. Although the competencies are seen as important for effective management of patients, they alone cannot deliver effective practice. There must be high-quality leadership within organisations and services to support staff in both service delivery and ongoing maintenance of their competency levels.

Table 3.1 Domains of Competency [8]

Domain A	Advanced clinical nursing practice
Domain B	Leading complex care co-ordination
Domain C	Proactively manage complex long-term conditions
Domain D	Managing cognitive impairment and mental well-being
Domain E	Supporting self-care, self-management and enabling independence
Domain F	Professional practice and leadership
Domain G	Identifying high-risk patients, promoting health and preventing ill health
Domain H	Managing care at the end of life
Domain I	Interagency and partnership working

The framework was developed from the evidence from pilot educational programmes for community matrons and case managers. The domains in the document are provided with indicative learning outcomes and the whole process is underpinned by some key principles without which the framework would not be successful. The principles include recognising prior learning, interprofessional learning, mentorship and coaching, assessment of competences, clinical supervision and continuing professional development. The ability to develop the framework in this way has added greatly to both its credibility and its effectiveness.

What the competencies are expected to deliver

The implementation of any new service in any area of care requires clear service aims and processes to ensure safe and effective delivery, case management is no different. The framework has assisted the development of services and enabled confidence in the professionals delivering the new services. The case management service model requires that staff to develop their abilities to support the transfer of responsibility from professionals to public in relation to self-care and monitoring. For staff to work in this way with any level of confidence, a supportive infrastructure including high levels of staff competency is required. If staff are confident and competent, they can work in an effective and safe way, thereby delivering high-quality care that meets the expectation of patients. The framework of competencies clearly outlines the skill set staff will use to facilitate this and all areas of intervention and support.

To accomplish the expected level of development in services, dramatic improvement is require in skills and competency. Although staff employed in current roles may have many skills and competencies, these are seen as requiring consolidation and expansion to enable safe service delivery. The competencies have been very effective and useful in service and staff development, but some of the professionals involved in managing patients with long-term needs feel the national focus has been overly biased to the higher level nursing skills. Despite this view, it is clear that in all of the other domains competencies are clearly transferable.

The competencies: what are they?

It is important at this stage to reflect in some detail on the competencies that have been developed for case managers and community matrons as the expectation is that a member of staff holding these competencies will deliver better outcomes for the patient. As explained earlier, each of the competencies has a number of subsets that allow learning outcomes and assessment of achievement and maintenance of competence to be completed. The subsets also allow staff to focus on their development needs in each domain as they may be able to evidence attainment in some area but not in the whole domain, which is to be expected as new staff commence in post.

Domain A: advanced clinical nursing practice

The clinical nursing skills are seen as those that will be utilised in active management of disease, particularly in relation to early recognition and management of deterioration in chronic conditions. These clinical skills, including prescribing, are fundamental in prevention of acute and emergency referral; the prevention of frequent emergency admissions is seen as a positive outcome for the patient. It is recognised that in some disease groups other professionals will also have many of the skills to recognise changes in disease patterns, particularly in relation to occupational therapy for rheumatoid disease and physiotherapy for some respiratory and vascular diseases. But in the main it is believed that the professionals with the highest capacity to deliver across all disease groups would be nurses, and this ability is advanced by the ability of the professionals to prescribe independently. Some allied health professionals can prescribe under supplementary prescribing arrangements, but currently only nurses and pharmacists can prescribe independently. Pharmacist can also prescribe independently but tend by experience to focus on single disease groups, though it is in no way beyond their skills to work across wider disease groups. Pharmacist may require extra clinical skills training as it is not routinely provided to the practitioners.

Within advanced nursing practice domain, the sub-competencies are as follows:

- Advanced clinical assessment skills;
- Advanced ability to assess and appropriately manage risk;
- Advanced ability to use information for undertaking assessments, clinical decision making and diagnosis;
- In-depth knowledge and understanding of the presentation, progression, pathophysiology and prognosis of common long-term conditions;
- In-depth knowledge and understanding of therapeutic interventions, including relevant pharmacology and medicines management;
- Advanced communication and interpersonal skills;
- In-depth knowledge of and ability to apply relevant legislation and full understanding of the ethical issues in caring for people with long-term conditions;
- Sophisticated application of holistic person-centred approaches to care.

The DH [10] outlines the advanced practitioner role and function and only those with who have achieved this level of competence are allowed to call themselves an advanced practitioner. The activities and abilities this advanced nursing practice competency allows are as follows:

- Ability to take a comprehensive history;
- Ability to carry out physical examinations;

- Ability to utilise expert knowledge and clinical judgement to identify a possible diagnosis;
- Confidence and ability to refer for investigation as appropriate;
- Ability to utilise all information to make a final diagnosis;
- Ability to make an informed clinical decision, decide and carry out appropriate treatment, including prescribing and referral to appropriate specialists;
- Ability to utilise extensive clinical expertise to plan and provide skilled and competent health and social care in partnership with other members of the healthcare team as appropriate;
- Ability to use expertise to ensure continuity of care through follow-up and review;
- Ability to utilise skills to review and evaluate the effectiveness of care and treatment with patients making amendments as appropriate;
- Capability and confidence to work independently, and also as part of a team;
- Experience and knowledge to act in a leadership role;
- Capability to ensure that all care delivered is based on best practice.

Currently, none of the other professional regulatory bodies have published anything similar in relation to advanced clinical practice definitions.

These purely clinical based competencies are those required within a community matron role and focus on the advanced clinical skills required to understand how disease progresses and its effect on the human body, what is normal and what is abnormal. These skills enable a practitioner to examine appropriately the systems in the body and utilise appropriate information to reach a diagnosis or clinical decision, and accordingly implement a care programme/treatment including pharmacological interventions. Once the treatment decision is made, a level of knowledge and understanding is required to review the decision and make changes. These types of competencies were for many years the domain of the medical profession and the development of these skills does require appropriate training and assessment to assure effective care and patient safety. These competencies will require clinical examination and diagnostic skills training and assessment underpinned by specific disease based knowledge and understanding and a through knowledge of therapeutic communication.

Subsets: advanced clinical assessment skills

This competence requires the practitioner to hold skills to assess, diagnose, prescribe and treat the patient. These skills are seen as those that enable assessment of clinical condition.

The subsets for this area are outlined in Table 3.2.

The other domains provided in the competency framework are applicable to all professionals working with those with long-term conditions. Each general domain and its possible impact on patient care and development processes is now outlined.

Table 3.2   Advanced Nursing Practice Subset Definitions of Ability

Subset	Definitions of ability
CMA1	The first of these requires the practitioner to be competent to obtain a medical history by completing a comprehensive data and information collection regarding history and examination. The practitioner will then be expected to interpret the findings and plan a programme of ongoing care in accordance to needs.
CMA2	This competence relates to the ability of the practitioner to assess and determine appropriately and effectively the functional ability and capacity of the patient and to make informed decisions on the processes of care required to ensure the management of these abilities.
CMA3	This competence relates to the ability of the practitioner to assess a patient with a chronic condition who presents with an altered health status. This will include making a diagnosis and managing the patient appropriately either personally or by referral to another practitioner. Competency is heavily reliant on the ability of the practitioner to examine the patient, analyse and interpret the findings and complete a risk assessment of the management options.
CMA4	This competence relates directly to the ability of a practitioner to assess, implement and monitor the care of a patient and their carers, ensuring ongoing effectiveness. The practitioner is expected to be able to use the competency to ensure agreement with patient and carers regarding ongoing care planning, including agreeing on nature of care and preparation for end-of-life care if appropriate.
CMA5	This competency requires that the practitioner is able to support the patients and carer to make choices in relation to patient care, working closely to assess needs and preferences and enabling, where possible, these to be delivered.
CMA6	This competence relates directly to medication management; medication issues are a high-risk area for patients with chronic diseases. It relates to the ability of the practitioner to understand and assess the medication patients are prescribed, and the patients' level of understanding and concordance with their medication. Monitoring of effectiveness and any side effects of medication is highly important.
CMA7	This competence is focused on the practice of prescribing medication to ensure the appropriate management of the patients' condition, and the practitioner must also be mindful of the Nursing and Midwifery Council Standards of Prescribing within this competency area.
CMPSL10	This competence relates to the practitioner holding and being able to utilise skills and knowledge to verify an expected death in line with local policies.

Domain B: leading complex care co-ordination

This domain focuses on that important area of care management which Americans call Care Orchestration – the ability in the practitioner to keep an overview of all care. The co-ordination function is fundamental to preventing many of the problems that occur for patients and their carers. Care co-ordination ensures effective levels of communication across the team involved in care and ensures that at all times the understanding of the patient's condition and management are clear.

One of the main problems for patients with long-term conditions is communication between primary and acute care. Despite sterling efforts, often communication delays cause major difficulties for patients in relation to repeat prescribing or other treatment plans. Poor communication particularly in relation to medication is a principal reason for readmission in many cases. The other area of poor communication that leads to problems for these patients relates to discharge from acute care. The provision of a safe and effective discharge from acute care requires excellent communication and also is assisted greatly by a 'key worker' who ensures all service can commence within an appropriate timescale and enables the patient to return home with confidence.

The ability of a case manager to manage and procure care for a patient with complex needs is also key to success as it is often only with excellent procurement and co-ordination that a level of independence can be maintained for some patients. A patient with complex needs will often be receiving care from a number of agencies and professional groups and the ability to ensure that this care is delivered effectively, and also in a resource appropriate way, can be a high wire act for the case manager; conflicting needs and expectations can cause problems for all involved.

The ability to act to protect patients at risk of abuse is also of key importance, as are excellent communication skills that enable the practitioner to develop a good therapeutic relationship with the patient and carers. The most effective case manager has a broad understanding of the services available within their area and knows how to access these effectively for the benefit of patients. They utilise statutory and third-sector services appropriately and ensure that those providing care and support are fully aware of the patient's needs and any changes in them.

The key areas to ensure these deliverables within this domain are as follows:

- Advanced ability to use and manage knowledge;
- In-depth knowledge and understanding of the health and well-being issues of people with long-term conditions;
- In-depth knowledge and understanding of and ability to manage interdisciplinary and team-based approaches to care;
- Knowledge and understanding of government policy and guidance on long-term conditions;
- Knowledge and understanding of service and resource procurement and management;
- Skills of identifying and protecting those at risk (particularly in relation to adult abuse), and caring for and supporting those individuals who have suffered abuse;
- Advanced communication and interpersonal skills;

- Sophisticated application of holistic person-centred approaches to care;
- In-depth knowledge of and ability to apply relevant legislation and full understanding of the ethical issues involved in caring for people with long-term conditions.

The subsets of this competency are defined in Table 3.3.

Table 3.3   Leading Complex Care Co-ordination Subset – Definitions of Ability

Subset	Definitions of ability
CMB1	This competency relates to the ability of a practitioner to plan, implement, monitor and review care plans and to ensure that care plans are personalised to the individual patient and carers needs and preferences. This will require an ability to identify when the care needs to be reviewed and changed and agree on this with the patient and carer.
CMB2	This competency relates to the ability of the practitioner to co-ordinate and review care across agencies and organisations and teams. The teams involved in care may be from a broad range of professional or nonprofessional backgrounds and may be well established or newly developed in response to the needs of the patient.
CMB3	This competence relates directly to patient safety. The practitioner must be able to robustly risk assess all care planning and decisions made to ensure that the patient is safe while supporting them to maintain independence.
CMB4	This competency relates directly to the ability of a practitioner to communicate in a variety of ways as appropriate to the patient needs and to maintain appropriate records, including ensuring appropriate sharing of records.
CMB5	This competence relates to the ability of the practitioner to identify the needs and preference of a patient and present these appropriately to ensure their wishes and preference are known, understood and acted upon.
CMB6	This competence relates to the ability of the practitioner to procure and access services to meet the needs of the patient. It is important in this competency for the practitioner to identify the requirements of the patient and then accordingly identify and contact for the appropriate services.
CMB7	This competency relates to the ability of a practitioner to utilise resources appropriately to both the needs of patients and the availability of those resources, while being mindful of the need to monitor the use of resources.
CMB8	This competence relates to the need for the practitioner to recognise and act upon any evidence of danger, harm or abuse to an individual. This competency needs to be viewed in line with local safeguarding vulnerable adults and children procedures.

Domain C: proactively manage complex long-term conditions

The next key domain relates to abilities to actually proactively manage complex long-term conditions. The key areas are as follows:

- Knowledge and understanding of the impact of socio-economic and personal circumstances on people with long-term conditions;
- In-depth knowledge and understanding of the impact of lifestyle choices on long-term conditions;
- Skills in managing clinical events, including risk assessment and appropriate management of risk;
- Advanced skills in managing and facilitating patients and carer education;
- In-depth knowledge and understanding of and ability to manage interprofessional and interagency working;
- In-depth knowledge and understanding of and ability to support the care of individuals in the home environment.

These skills and competencies are clearly aimed at ensuring the effective ongoing assessment and management of chronic conditions and their impacts on patients. The ability to support patients in understanding and managing their own conditions is fundamental to the maintenance of independence and choice for these patients and their carers. These skills will ensure that the case manager is able to plan or at least assess the trajectory of the patient's disease and understand what, if any, further complications and problems may occur next. These skills will also enable the case manager to recognise what can and should be delivered within a home environment, how the safety of this care can be assured and how to minimise and manage any potential risks. The type of issues that could be managed by these skills is the presence of oxygen in a house with fires or smokers.

Table 3.4 outlines the key areas of competence within the subsets.

Domain D: managing cognitive impairment and mental well-being

Patients with long-term conditions are more likely to suffer from depression and anxiety than the 'healthy population' and as many of these patients are in the older age groups, they are also more likely to develop problems with cognitive impairment. Mental well-being is a highly important but not well-managed issue in general terms, therefore, all case managers will need to develop very early the ability to assess the mental well-being and cognitive abilities. The latter is particularly relevant in relation to choice and consent to care and treatment processes, as is a clear understanding of the ethical and legal issues relating to long-term care and mental capacity. For many professionals, this is the most difficult and

Table 3.4 Proactively Manage Complex Long Term Conditions Subset – Definitions of Ability

Subset	Definition of ability
CMC1	This competency relates to the practitioners' ability to develop practices that enable choice, well-being and protection, including planning, monitoring and reviewing care plans.
CMC2	This competency relates to assessment skills utilised by the practitioner either initially on admission to the caseload or as a follow-up, which will lead to a care plan that is agreed by the patient and carer. This care plan may relate to particular actions relating to behaviour change required by the patient.
CMC3	This competence relates to the ability of the practitioner to support and empower the patient to make choices in relation to their health and well-being. This competency is supported through the newly published NHS Constitution [11] in relation to promoting the rights and responsibilities of individuals to make decisions for themselves as appropriate, supported by professionals in this process.
CMC4	This competency relates to the ability of the practitioner to identify the needs and to enable and support the patients to live independently within their home, including the identification of appropriate changes to the environment.
CMC5	This competency relates to building partnerships with patients, carers and team members, being mindful at all time of the role everyone plays in enabling and supporting the patients. The practitioner should be able to identify the roles required to enable the delivery of the care plan and then ensure delivery of those roles to improve the health and social outcomes for the patient.
CMC6	This competency relates directly to the management of the care team, ensuring safety and security.

challenging area of skills development as knowledge relating to mental health is often seen as a specialist skill; despite this, many case managers have developed these skills effectively.

The competency subsets are as follows:

- Knowledge and understanding of sources of information on mental health and related services;
- Skills in the assessment of mental health needs, including risk assessment;
- Knowledge and understanding of physical, behavioural, emotional and psychological indications of mental health needs;
- Knowledge and understanding of counselling and psychological support methods;
- Skills in interpreting responses to long-term conditions including recognition of the signs of depression;
- In-depth knowledge and understanding of diversity, discrimination and stigmatisation;

- Knowledge and understanding of therapeutic interventions;
- Advanced communication and interpersonal skills.

Table 3.5 outlines the key areas of competence within the subsets.

Table 3.5   Managing Cognitive Impairment and Mental Wellbeing Subset – Definitions of Ability

Subset	Definition of ability
CMD1	This competency relates directly to the skills required for the initial identification of mental health needs. The practitioner is required to identify and act on evidence of mental health needs.
CMD2	This competency relates to the ability of practitioners to refer into mental health services in a timely and appropriate way.
CMD3	This competency relates to the need for practitioners to contribute to the assessment, planning, evaluation and review of individualised programmes of care for individuals. This would include utilisation of a broad range of assessment and review tools as appropriate to the patient needs.
CMD4	This competency relates to the practitioners ability to implement specific parts of a programme of care as part of a wider team working with a co-ordinated team approach in a way that has been agreed with the patient.
CMD5	This competency relates to the ability of a practitioner to identify and provide or refer for psychological support for the patient or carers as required. This competency requires the development of a co-ordinated response to the needs of patients and carers within and across teams.
CMD6	This competency relates to the practitioners ability to develop and enable carers and all other support networks to care or support an individual to maintain independence and live in their own home. These networks could include a wide variety of persons including family, friends and religious leaders.
CMD7	This competence relates directly to how a practitioner will support and empower patients and their carers to represent their views and organise their own care through direct payments etc.
CMD8	This competency relates to how the practitioner enables and encourages patients to maintain involvement in social and other networks and activities that will improve independence and social well-being.
CMD9	This competency relates to the processes and skills the practitioner utilises to ensure that patients with long-term conditions are treated in an equitable and fair way and are included within mainstream cultural and other activities. This competency links directly to both health inequalities in relation to service access and to equality and diversity legislation.

Domain E: supporting self-care, self-management and enabling independence

Throughout all chronic disease intervention models self-care and independence are key principles. All recent NHS policy drivers clearly outline the expectation that services will focus on enabling patients' to be empowered to self-care, implement behavioural change to improve their health and make informed choices about their care. The NHS Constitution [12] reinforces this by describing for the public what they can expect from the NHS and what the NHS can expect in return. Working with the public to develop their capacity and capability to manage their own health either in relation to lifestyles and behaviours or in relation to minor and chronic disease is extremely challenging. The NHS since its inception has told the public that 'if you are ill we will look after you' and while that remains the case, we know from public health data that the lifestyle behaviours of many people are having significant long-term impacts on their health.

The ability to work with patients and their carers and to identify their levels of understanding and the information they need and want in a way that is understandable and acceptable is an essential skill in all areas of health. In relation to prevention of disease from a population perspective, it is clear that multiple methods of information and education are needed. Once patients are diagnosed with a long-term condition, a whole new set of challenges develop. Dependent on a number of factors, responses to the news of their diagnosis and their ongoing ability to understand and self-manage their disease will range from almost none engagement to easy acceptance and concordance with advice and of course all points in between. The ability to understand your long-term condition is fundamental to your ability to cope with its impact and have an element of control. Some patients are more able than others in this regard, but as the amount of time a patient spends with a professional carer is probably less than 3 hours in a year, they need to understand at least at some level their disease. It is clearly reported by patients that the more they understand, the more in control and the better they feel, and it should be noted that patients almost always know themselves best.

Supporting self-care is also about promoting and enabling independence. For some years, the number of patients admitted to long-term care has been on the rise. This is obviously not acceptable as with appropriate support some of these patients, if it is their wish, could be maintained in their own home. Local authorities in partnership with the NHS have been given challenging targets to increase the number of patients living in a supported way at home through the use of telemedicine and support. To make these support processes work, patients and carers must trust the professionals and the equipment, and the only way to deliver this is by ensuring that all involved understand what the support does and how it will work in practical terms. The patients and carers also need to understand the boundaries in which they can manage themselves to reduce the amount of risk and to ensure appropriate responses are always provided.

The key subsets are as follows:

- Skills in partnership with patients and carers;
- Knowledge, understanding and application of cognitive behavioural therapy techniques;
- Advanced conflict and dispute management skills;
- In-depth knowledge and understanding of community resources and support networks;
- Advanced skills in empowering patients and enabling self-care;
- In-depth knowledge and understanding of self-advocacy;
- In-depth knowledge and understanding of the impact of long-term conditions on everyday life;
- Knowledge and understanding of individual rights;
- Advanced teaching and coaching skills;
- In-depth knowledge and understanding of the impact of lifestyle choices on long-term conditions.

Table 3.6 outlines the key areas of competence within the subsets.

Table 3.6 Supporting Self Care, Self Management and Enabling Independence Subsets – Definitions of Ability

Subset	Definition of ability
CME1	This competency relates to the need for practitioners to be skilled in assessing the need for behavioural change and encouraging and empowering change to promote health, improve the quality of life and reduce complications.
CME2	This competency outlines the need for the practitioner to be able to support patients to evaluate and assess the appropriateness and effectiveness of support structures, be they formal or informal, and to support and enable patients to utilise these appropriately.
CME3	This competency outlines the need for the practitioner to be able to support patients to evaluate and assess the appropriateness and effectiveness of support structures in relation to assistive devices and technology.
CME4	This competency recognises the need for practitioner involved in care of patients with chronic conditions to be able to support and enable patients to undertake occupational, leisure and other everyday activities.
CME5	This competency relates to the ability of the practitioner to support patients cope and manage the impact of their long-term health problems on their day-to-day functioning, engaging with appropriate support structures.
CMEL11	This competency relates to the practitioner's abilities in relation to teaching learners, including carers and patients, to use equipment or carry out procedures or care through demonstration or instruction.
CMEL12	This competency relates to how the practitioner will use coaching skills to support learning for carers and patients.
CMEL13	This competence relates directly to the needs for practitioners to be effective teachers to groups including their teams, so the competency requires the practitioner to understand group dynamics and the impact these have on effective learning and when group learning is an appropriate learning model to use.

Domain F: professional practice and leadership

All professionals will have somewhere within their professional codes a require-ment to act as a leader in a team, service or the profession and to be mindful of the perception of their actions. Leadership in the context of case management is very clearly a case of leading the charge in services for quality and safety, but the role model function as the leader of a care team is also highly important. Professional practice can be defined as acting at all times in an appropriate way, which is in line with the appropriate professional code.

Another key principle is ensuring at all times that actions taken are within the practitioners level of competence and also, if a duty is delegated, that the person to which the duty is delegated is capable and competent. This area of competence would require the practitioner to understand how they would assess the level of competence of a team member and how they would ensure that any lacking competency is developed through appraisal and training. This area of competence would include the need to ensure that the practitioners have personally received appropriate development for their role and that their team is also appropriately trained and skilled. All registered professionals are accountable and responsible for their actions and must ensure that their acts or omissions never place a patient at risk and are always in the best interest of a patient.

Professional practice and leadership competencies are essential in ensuring governance and quality in services, and all case managers would be required to work within appropriate governance structures and clinical guidelines. They are also required to maintain their own skills and competencies through continuing professional development. There is an important requirement within this domain for the use of and support of clinical supervision for all practitioners; clinical supervision is seen in this context as essential to support practitioners working with highly complex patients who are often very ill and will require extensive support. Clinical supervision will enable peer review and support structure and probably enable practice reflection to improve practice.

The key subsets are as follows:

- In-depth knowledge and understanding of professional accountability;
- In-depth knowledge and understanding of workforce development, profes-sional development, supervision and appraisal;
- Highly developed reflective practice skills;
- In-depth knowledge and understanding of relevant clinical governance issues;
- Advanced leadership skills;
- In-depth knowledge and understanding of organisational development and change management;
- In-depth knowledge and understanding of the issues relating to personal and professional competence.

Table 3.7 outlines the key areas of competence within the subsets.

Table 3.7   Professional Practice and Leadership Subsets – Definitions of Ability

Subset	Definition of ability
CMF1	This competency relates to the practitioners requirement to act as a clinical lead within the care team and to ensure the continuing development of the team, through sharing of knowledge and supervision, and of themselves, through review of competency and recognition of areas for development.
CMF2	This competency requires the practitioner to promote the values and principles that enable the delivery of best practice in all care areas, including legislation and care guidelines. This relates directly to the need to maintain knowledge and skills and to continuously develop professionally and personally.
CMF3	This competency relates directly to the ability of the practitioners as professionals to work within their level of competence and to ensure that the care and processes delivered are in line with protocols and guidelines agreed with their employers. A key area in this competency is the need for the practitioners to recognise clearly their level of responsibility and accountability.
CMF4	This competency relates to the need for practitioners to provide leadership within their employing organisation to lead the development of policy and procedure to ensure effective and safe practice for patients.
CMF5	This competency relates to the need for practitioners to develop, sustain and evaluate all areas of collaborative work, facilitating delivery and ensuring patients are cared for appropriately.

Domain G: identifying high-risk people, promoting health and preventing ill health

This domain provides for the skills and abilities required within the case manager to identify appropriate very high intensity users and ways in which their health and well-being can be promoted.

The key subsets are as follows:

- Skills in analysing, interpreting and presenting public health data;
- Knowledge and understanding of evaluation methodologies and associated ethics;
- In-depth knowledge and understanding of social constructions of health and illness.

These competencies relate very clearly to the ability of case managers and their services to identify the appropriate patients to manage. But they also include skills that enable a full understanding of the impact of long-term conditions socially and from a public health perspective. The way society reacts to those with long-term conditions affects directly how they view themselves in the world and their ability to function as an individual. The level of chronic disease and disability has an important impact on the community, and it is very

Table 3.8 Identifying High Risk People, Promoting Health and Preventing Ill Health Subsets – Definitions of Ability

Subset	Definitions of ability
CMG1	This competency relates to the ability of a practitioner to work in partnership with colleagues, including public health, to identify and analyse the health needs of a specific population, including the potential stressors on the population that will affect detrimentally the health and well-being of the population. This will include health protection issues including vaccination status and uptake.
CMG2	This competency relates to the skills used by the practitioner to communicate the information relating to health and well-being in the population. The information may be communicated to case find or manage the population, thereby improving health.
CMG3	This competency relates to the sharing and presenting of information in relation to health and well-being of the caseload to enable surveillance, health planning, health protection and improved choice.
CMG4	This competency relates to the skills and expertise required in the practitioner to enable them to communicate effectively with individuals, groups and communities to promote their health and well-being.
CMG5	This competency relates to how the practitioner will work in partnership to protect the health and well-being of the population; this could include prevention of infection etc.
CMG6	This competency relates to the abilities of a practitioner to improve health and well-being of their caseload working in partnership with communities.

clear from public health data that levels of chronic disease are higher in many deprived areas. It is also clear that the level of health inequality in an area will directly impact on the ability of service to respond to identified need. All professionals working in health and social care are expected to support the delivery of strong public health messages, particularly those that relate to poor health behaviours that would impact on the prevalence of long-term conditions and of course the progress of disease.

Table 3.8 outlines the key areas of competence within the subsets.

Domain H: end-of-life care

No matter what the process of care is, all chronic diseases will eventually owing to either disease progression or complications and co-morbidity require end-of-life care. The delivery of palliative care for those patients with cancer is well established via pathways for symptom control. The main problem with those diseases that are seen as life limiting is that it is often difficult for professionals to admit that the time has been reached when palliation is the most appropriate management plan.

Table 3.9 End of Life Care Subsets – Definitions of Ability

Subset	Definition of ability
CMH1	This competency relates to the requirement for the practitioner to support in an effective and appropriate way patients and carers who are experiencing significant life events. This could include loss or major changes.
CMH2	This competency relates to the practitioners' ability to support individuals through bereavement and help them manage the changes bereavement causes.
CMH3	This competency relates to the practitioners' ability to care and support patients and carers at the end of life, including appropriately managing symptoms and enabling choice and preferred place of care.

Palliative care teams are now developing their skills in many chronic diseases, particularly respiratory disease and heart failure, where patients can spend a substantial part of the end of their life with difficult to manage symptoms such as breathlessness. It is absolutely essential that case managers are able to recognise the changes and deterioration in conditions to ensure delivery of appropriate support and management of symptoms. It is also important that practitioners are competent and able to provide appropriate support when decision to manage symptoms for comfort rather than improvement is made. This can be a difficult decision and of course discussion for patients, carers and practitioners, but it is a discussion that needs to take place to ensure and enable patients and their carers to make appropriate choices and plans for the care at the end of life.

The key subsets are as follows:

- Knowledge and understanding of life stages and changes and losses associated with long-term conditions;
- Knowledge and understanding of how individuals respond to distress;
- Skills in the care of the dying and bereavement care.

Table 3.9 outlines the key areas of competence within the subsets.

Domain I: interagency and partnership working

This final domain is that in which the case manager will be collaborating, negotiating and influencing service provision. The delivery of care to those with long-term conditions requires robust partnerships and collaboration to enable effective outcomes. In the provision of care to those with chronic diseases, there is never a time when collaboration with a partner (another agency, a carer, the patient or another professional) is not a requirement. It is essential that a case manager can

Table 3.10   Interagency and Partnership Working Subsets – Definitions of Ability

Subset	Definition of ability
CMI1	This competency outlines the skills required within the practitioners to enable effective management of the caseload. The management of the caseload must ensure the best possible outcomes for the patients, by ensuring that all care is designed to promote and achieve the best possible outcomes.
CMI2	This competency applies to those practitioners who do not have line management responsibilities but will be required to manage and evaluate performance of teams in other agencies to ensure effective and appropriate services to individual patients.
CMI3	This competency relates to those practitioners who will be facilitating and enabling discharge or transfer between services and highlights the skills required to ensure safe and effective discharge and transfer including clear and agreed discharge planning and communication with carers and agencies.
CMI4	This competency is key for the practitioner as it outlines the skills required to ensure the delivery of effective partnerships in the provision of care, and includes agreements in relation to boundaries, roles and responsibilities in joint working.

evidence high levels of skills in this arena as integration across care is the only way that provision can deliver at all the levels required to meet the patients' needs.

The key subsets are as follows:

- In-depth knowledge and understanding of collaborative and interagency working;
- Knowledge and understanding of performance review;
- Advanced conflict and dispute management skills;
- Advanced communication and interpersonal skills.

Table 3.10 outlines the key areas of competence within the subsets.

What the competencies aim to do

The competencies are clearly developed to enable patient care and ensure safety, but they also aim to provide to practitioners a clear set of parameters against which they can assess themselves in preparation for a case management post or while in post for ongoing professional development.

It is clear that across the domains a number of key competencies are repeated, communication and interpersonal skills, dispute management, negotiation, partnership and collaboration to name but a few. It is also clear that many of the skills required would be present in all professionals within the workforce. The DH educational framework required that organisations utilised the tool to identify how they would ensure that the case managers and community matrons employed are fit for purpose and capable of delivering the required outcomes for patients.

A number of organisations across the NHS worked with the framework to develop educational processes to support the development of these competencies in their case managers. The framework CD provides an overview of how they completed these processes. The only absolute guidance from the department in this area was that the advanced clinical roles (community matrons) were probably nursing roles and that all case managers must have the ability to study at master's level. This latter guidance has caused some discussion and led to slightly different levels of interpretation. In some areas, the response of organisations has been that all staff must have a master's level qualification or be working towards. Some organisations have taken a more pragmatic view and decided that if the case manager can complete successfully a programme of level 4 education, designed to provide the education needed to cover all the competencies within the framework, then that is sufficient preparation.

Developing educational models to develop competencies

Cheshire and Merseyside Strategic Health Authority made the latter decision and in collaboration with all their local higher educational institutions developed a three-module, 60-credit Post-Graduate Diploma in Managing Long-Term Conditions. The programme modules included guidelines for clinical and diagnostic skills, therapeutic communication and professional practice and managing long-term conditions [13]. This programme provided to all those staff employed in case management or community matron roles an education process to develop the skills required. The programme was delivered using a blended learning approach and in line with the national education framework, which allowed for staff to use their prior learning as a starter point with which they could assess their personal learning needs. The national framework while providing the competencies and very detailed advice on what these competencies mean in real terms for the practitioner is very clear that previous experience and experiential learning must be recognised within the process of assessing educational and developmental needs. The key process in developing and maintaining competencies for case managers is the use of expert mentors and professional networks of case managers to enable sharing of experience and expertise. The ability of practitioners to develop and maintain clinical networks for peer support is reported anecdotally by practitioners as providing high levels of support and assists in the development of confidence within roles both during education and post education. Cheshire and Merseyside strategic authority competed as part of their processes to support the implementation of case management within their area a stock-take of the long-term conditions workforce in December 2006 [13], which highlighted some wide differences in workforce preparedness for case management and in preparedness of organisations to implement safely and effectively case management models of care.

Essex workforce development confederation [8] also utilised this framework, but they decided to use the process to identify clearly the overall development needs of their workforce rather than just those in relation to chronic diseases and case management. The decision was made that by commissioning an integrated workforce development programme they could deliver not only the high-priority long-term conditions agenda but also workforce modernisation. The plans for implementation of education programmes in Essex included a high level of commitment from the medical consultants who were involved in the assessment and support of all case managers completing the development programme. This support was seen as essential in ensuring the credibility of the staff and the confidence of the medics in the training.

In the Midlands, Birmingham and the Black Country, health economy worked together to develop an educational programme for case managers. The programme is of 1 year in length and at completion the case manager will hold a post-graduate certificate in advanced practice. The programme has been developed like many of the others in collaboration across higher education institutions and providers to ensure the development of staff who are fit for purpose.

Whatever the training process for case managers to develop these competencies, an assessment of prior learning and knowledge is very important to enable the development process to focus on the areas of the most need. Many of the staff who enter case management roles and then undertake these programmes are already highly skilled and experienced and it is important that training and development is delivered to meet a development need and not just because a practitioner has been recruited to the role. Having said this, it is clear that all those who have completed the development and educational programmes designed by organisations have gained enormously from the experience. It is also fair to say that the delivery of development programmes whether inhouse or via higher educational establishments is reliant on excellent mentorship and clinical support. All areas that developed programmes have provided this support alongside the educational and other support. The ability of mentors, usually medical colleagues, to support the development particularly of clinical skills does enable a high level of credibility and confidence in the staff when they complete programmes, as the process is seen to have an appropriate level of rigour.

Those organisations that have not designed stand-alone programmes of development have used the framework and the tools within it to assess the competence of staff at recruitment or during personal development processes. This assessment of knowledge and prior learning and experience has enabled effective identification of gaps in knowledge, which have then been managed via inhouse and other developmental programmes. The process for assessment of competency must be robust as without this the credibility of the professionals involved would be negatively affected and patient safety may be compromised. The DH framework encourages organisations to develop robust governance processes for both recruitment and staff review as this is seen as the most effective way of ensuring safe outcomes for patients.

Evaluation of educational and developmental programmes for case managers is in progress in many places across the NHS. The evaluations are reviewing the effectiveness of the education programmes in relation to confidence and competence of staff, patient safety (untoward incident numbers), achievement of expected outcomes, views of medical and other colleagues and of course views of patients and carers. There is no doubt that early pilot sites for case management where these evaluations have already been completed were able to show some very positive outcomes for staff and patients. The level of confidence and competence in most staff was very high and their clinical skills were maintained at a high level by ongoing mentorship and peer support. The outcomes and satisfaction for patients in these areas appear to be fairly good with positive feedback on confidence levels and feelings of high levels of support and management.

Conclusion

The development of competencies for case management models and the professionals to deliver this was a key policy of the DH in relation to the management of long-term conditions. Patients with long-term conditions are vulnerable and have highly complex needs and require care delivered by highly skilled and experienced practitioners. The competency outline and its underpinning educational framework provided essential tools in delivering the skilled practitioners required. It is essential that practitioners are competent, and assessment against formal competency frameworks provides assurance for patients and of course employers. Competency frameworks are important in all areas of professional practice and are essential in area where professionals are potentially working in advanced practice, providing a clear safety net to ensure practitioners are 'fit for purpose'.

References

1. World Health Organisation (1998). *Learning to Work Together for Health: Report of a World Health Organisation Study Group on Multiprofessional Education for Health Personnel: A Team Approach.* http://www.who.int/publications/en/(accessed on October 2009).
2. Eraut M (2001). *Keynote Paper at the Fifth International Conference on the Regulation of Nursing and Midwifery.* (www.rcn.org.uk)
3. Royal College of Nursing and Parkinson's Disease Society (2005). *Competences: An Integrated Career and Competency Framework for Nurses Working in Parkinson's Disease Management.* http://www.rcn.org.uk/_data/assets/pdf_file/0005/156164/003065.pdf
4. Department of Health (1998). *Making a Difference: Strengthening the Nursing, Midwifery and Health Visiting Contribution to Health and Healthcare.* http://www.dh.gov.uk/prod_consum_dh/groups/dh_digitalassets/@dh/@en/documents/digitalasset/dh_4074704.pdf (accessed on October 2009).
5. NHS Executive (1999). *Agenda for Change.* http://www.dh.gov.uk/prod_consum_dh/groups/dh_digitalassets/@dh/@en/documents/digitalasset/dh_4099423.pdf (accessed on October 2009).

6. Benner P (1984). *From Novice to Expert: Excellence and Power in Clinical Nursing Practice*. Addison Wesley Publishing Sacremento.
7. NHS Executive (2001). *Report of the Enquiry into Bristol Royal Infirmary*. http://www.bristol-inquiry.org.uk/final_report/report/index.htm (accessed on October 2009).
8. NHS Executive (2000). *Report of the External Review into Oxford Cardiac Service*. http://www.dh.gov.uk/prod_consum_dh/groups/dh_digitalassets/@dh/@en/documents/digitalasset/dh_4100718.pdf (accessed on October 2009).
9. Department of Health (2006). *Caring for People with Long Term Conditions: An Education Framework for Community Matrons and Case Managers*. http://www.dh.gov.uk/prod_consum_dh/groups/dh_digitalassets/@dh/@en/documents/digitalasset/dh_4118102.pdf (accessed on October 2009).
10. NHS Modernisation Agency and Skills for Health (2005). *Knowledge and Skills for Managing Long Term Conditions*. http://www.healthcareworkforce.nhs.uk/resources/latest_resources/long_term_neurological_conditions.html
11. National Workforce Projects (2005). *UK Wide Workforce Planning Competency Framework*. http://www.healthcareworkforce.nhs.uk/capabilityandcapacity.html (accessed on October 2009).
12. Department of Health (January 2009). *NHS Constitution*. http://www.dh.gov.uk/prod_consum_dh/groups/dh_digitalassets/documents/digitalasset/dh_093442.pdf (accessed on October 2009).
13. Cheshire & Merseyside Strategic Health Authority (December 2006). *Stock-Take of Long Term Conditions Workforce Development*. Report to the Long Term Conditions Programme Board (www.cheshireandmerseysideshs.nhs.uk)

Chapter 4
Outcomes for Patients – Managing Complex Care

Introduction

Effectiveness of case management is reliant on the case manager utilising all appropriate competencies to achieve best possible outcome for the patient. This chapter reviews the potential impacts of three specific competency sets. Although it needs to be understood that competencies will not be used in isolation, the concept is to look at what each specific competency means in terms of delivery for patients and their carers/support networks. Case management services have been developed to deliver some specific service outcomes, but broader patient benefits are possible and their measurement is essential. This chapter reviews domains B, G and I in some detail to reflect possible and expected impacts on patients and carers.

The outcomes on patients from the areas of competencies reviewed in this chapter focus in the main on those skills that deliver assessment of need, planning of care and organisation of care delivery for either individuals or case loads. These competencies are not purely skills delivered via nursing roles but those that are held by all professionals involved in long-term care. For each area of competence, the performance criteria are reviewed and the actual outcomes they can potentially deliver are described [1]. Some areas are reviewed in detail to outline their importance on outcomes.

The areas of competence and deliverables for patients: Leading complex care co-ordination

Competency B1

This competency set describes the need for the case manager to work with individuals and carers to plan, implement, monitor and review care plans developed for individual patients and their carers. The ability to deliver this competence requires that the professional develops an effective relationship with the individual to agree the roles and responsibilities of their carers. This requirement enables the professional to clearly understand how the carer is to be involved in the delivery of care and to understand the level of support the carer will need to deliver the agreed role. Carers carry for their relatives an enormous pressure of care that they deliver in place of health and social care. The level of care provided by these 'informal care arrangements' enables many patients to remain independently in their homes and reduces the financial burden on the state. Case managers are seen as highly effective in supporting carers and reducing the stresses and pressures of care responsibilities [2].

It is essential to have the ability to communicate in appropriate ways with patients and carers to ensure a full understanding of the disease process, any interventions and plans for their care, including the advice on effective management of the disease, or disability, including process for early recognition of deterioration and what actions to take. This competence is important in terms of ensuring not only consent but also safety of the patient. The ability of service users and carers to make informed decision on how their services are provided requires that they understand impacts and outcomes of the decision they make.

Communication skills are also fundamental to the ability of practitioners to provide information to service users and carers in relation to care plans. For service users and carers to agree plans they must understand clearly what these plans mean for them, what the care delivery will be, how they will access support when needed and how the effectiveness of the care will be monitored. Identification of information that is easily accessible and understandable is an essential part of the communication and negotiation process. Unless the individual understands what the plan is how can they effectively agree with its delivery, comply with the plan and the actions they need to take as part of the plan or feel confident enough to access assistance when required. Individuals in receipt of care and their support networks must feel confident in the plan and those delivering care, as through this they will achieve an appropriate level of independence and self-care that is impossible in any other arrangement.

The ability of patients to make informed decisions and thereby provide consent is both a human right and a legal requirement [3]. To ensure and enable informed consent is also a professional requirement; all professional codes require that the registrants act appropriately to ensure informed consent. For the older people the need for protection from possible abuse and any potential loss of their human rights because of vulnerability has been highlighted as highly important and has led to calls for a clearly defined set of rights for patients [4]. This has been promoted and delivered through the NHS Constitution [5] that clearly outlines all the responsibilities and expectations for both staff and users of the NHS.

The practitioner should have the ability to negotiate and discuss the areas of disagreement so that the individuals and carers accept the plan of care. The perspectives and views that individuals have on care should be understood and respected by the professional. The ability to respect any individuals' needs and expectations even if they appear to be at odds with their best interests is an essential requirement if we are to ensure that services are truly delivered in with the patient as the central point for organisation. Help the Aged have produced some clear definitions of how patients would wish to be treated, and respect is highlighted as an important issue for older people [6].

The practitioner should work in a partnership with individuals and carers to identify their preferences for care, including timing, location and frequency. If services are not able to deliver the preferences of individual and their carers, then the practitioner must be able to communicate and negotiate a delivery process that is acceptable to them. Increased patient choice and provision of care closer to home as outlined in current policy documents for the NHS, including the NHS review [7], enables patients to choose care services that provide them with care where and when they need it. The models of care that are viewed as designed for the benefit of providers of care rather than users are no longer acceptable. The patients expect that care services will provide relief in the way they want. Although this is not always possible, it is important that case managers as orchestrators of care act as advocate for individuals and carers challenging models of care that do not deliver in the way individuals require.

A key competence for case managers is the ability to build the confidence of individuals and carers to take an active role in their own care and in managing their disease, taking actions that promote health and well-being. This would help all individuals to take actions to improve their own and their families' health behaviours.

All outcomes in this area for individuals and carers relate to the ability to be involved and choose the care processes that they are comfortable with and that deliver in a safe and legal way what they feel they need. Positive outcomes for users of care are that they are empowered, are confident of care delivery and feel in control. These have been identified in many of the reviews of case management [2]. Professional outcomes in this area relate to professional practice and their ability to effectively influence and negotiate through information and communication.

Competency B2

This competency relates to the ability of the practitioner to coordinate care to meet the needs of individuals across multiple agencies. Professionals involved in case management must be able to communicate effectively across a broad range of teams to ensure that care delivery is safe and effective and of course in line with the individuals needs. Practitioners are required by their professional code to ensure the safety of care through robust and appropriate communication and information sharing. While information sharing must be in line with legal requirements, it must also ensure that individuals are not at risk.

When plans for care are agreed with individuals and carers, these agreements must be appropriately communicated to care team members to ensure and enable delivery. Only through clear information sharing can teams deliver safe and effective care. This process of information sharing will also enable effective monitoring of care delivery and will enable review and updating of plans as required if goals and objectives agreed with individuals and carers have not been or are not being achieved. Reviews and evaluations of care planning require practitioners to record in a robust and clear way any amendments or changes to the planned care agreed with individuals or carers and teams. The information on changes must be communicated immediately to ensure effective services are provided.

It is essential to have the ability to deliver in an appropriate way the competencies in this area, provide outcomes for individuals and carers in relation to safe and effective care in line with their requirements and ensure that staff understand the expectations on them. These levels of understanding should reduce risks in relation to complaints and will provide all involved with defined processes for care that should ensure the quality of the interventions.

Competency B3

This competency focusses on the support enabling individuals to live independently through reduction and management of risk. For most individuals with long-term care needs, the key is to maintain independence within their own home, to do this there are times when a level of risk needs to be taken. Risk is inherent in everything we do; every decision we make in our daily lives is in effect influenced by some form of understanding of the risk in the decision. For people who are fit and well, risks are managed at an individual level and relate specifically to their own actions. For those with long-term health or care needs, risk is different. In this situation understanding of risk must include knowledge of their specific disease or health need, how this will progress and what can be reasonably expected.

The ability to assess and manage risk in case management requires that the practitioner can understand in detail, not only how the individual is now, but also how they have been and how their health or care need may progress in the future. This requires high levels of knowledge of specific health needs and how these progress. This also requires high-level skills that allow the practitioner to communicate this understanding to individuals and carers. The skills will also include an ability to explain and debate with the user of service and carers levels of potential risk and how these can be mitigated. Individuals must understand risk and impact to allow them to make appropriate decisions and to ensure they can understand how these can be managed or when things do go wrong this can be recognised early and action taken. Risk issues could include security of the environment, utilisation of equipment, changes in clinical conditions, vulnerability, falls risks, medication, moving and handling. There will be times when a risk requires specialist assessment and the practitioner must be able to recognise their limitations in these areas. Risks could affect individuals and carers both professional and informal. Risks must be understood and managed; this is not about risk aversion it is about being risk aware to enable care, and when an unacceptable risk is identified an appropriate action is taken to prevent the risk. The outcomes for service users and carers (formal and informal) in this area are focused on ensuring safety and supporting decision making to enable independence.

Competency B4

This competency area is very much focused on the ability of case managers to develop and use processes and systems of communication, including recording and reporting. The performance criteria outline the requirements of the case manager in relation to communication with patients and carers, and with professionals and colleagues internally and externally.

The outcomes expected and delivered for this domain for patients and carers are related to the ability of the case manager to support them to communicate in a way that is effective for them. It is clear that communication and the ability to have views and preferences understood are essential for patients and carers. The case manager should be able to utilise appropriate skills to identify barriers to good communication and work to facilitate/enable communication. An immediate issue to be assessed by the case manager must be the communication requirements of patients and their carers. The ability to recognise difficulties when they arise and take appropriate action to enable effective communication cannot be underestimated. This is important not just for the case manager but also for all service providing staff.

The ability to recognise the range of communication models and processes that may be required is essential. Patients and carers should be treated at all times in line with all equalities legislation, and the ability of professionals to enable communication models is an important part of the care process. To deliver person-centred care, as required in all recent policy guidance [5,7] including the delivery of choice, professionals and care providers should be able to share information with patients and carers in a way that is both effective and appropriate to their needs.

Patients and carers can present with a range of communication needs. Evaluations of case management such as the Evercare Review [2] have outlined that the ability to assess the communication needs and be flexible in models of communication is valued highly. The broad range of communication needs cannot be underestimated and the ability to recognise when specialist advice or support is needed to enable communication is an essential skill. It can be easy to assess communication problems in some patients groups and their carers, for example, if a person is registered blind this is often recorded in referral information, but this is not always the case with literacy. It is not acceptable for communication in any form to be provided if the provider of the information is not sure that the receiver can understand its presentation. Professionals while very caring do occasionally forget that for patients and carers, the language and jargon used is highly complex and potentially may mean nothing to them.

A case manager should act as a role model in this area. He or she must work with providers, both internal and external, to ensure that everyone involved has an understanding of the communication needs of the patient and carer. The most valued services to patients and carers are those that treat them with dignity and respect [8], and it is without doubt that the ability to communicate appropriately is one of the frameworks that enables and ensures this occurs.

Communication should be effective. Evaluation of how effective a communication is can be highly complex as it will depend on the expectation of the communication. For effective communication with patients and carers we should understand their expectations of the communication alongside the expectations we hold as professionals. Effective communication for patients and carers is that which provides them with the information and knowledge they require or request to make a decision on what happens to them, or to understand a decision that may be made on their behalf. The communication models used will depend on the information being supplied and the presentation style preferred by the patient and carer; therefore, professionals must use a communication model that is 'fit for purpose'.

Effective communication is also affected by robust record-keeping. All professionals are required by their registration body (Nursing and Midwifery Council, Health Professions Council, General Medical Council, etc.) and national legal requirements to maintain accurate and contemporaneous records. This requirement is clearly outlined in all professional codes, and all NHS and social care guidance has also set out clear expectations in relation to record-keeping [9,10]. Recording essential and appropriate information ensures patient and staff safety. Clear reporting reduces the risk of errors in delivery of care. It is expected that patients will have full access to their records. All case management services utilise patient–held records that the patient and carer have been involved in development of and will often have signed up to care plans. A very positive outcome for users of case management service in all evaluations is that increased understanding and ownership of care planning enables personal choice.

Competency B5

This area relates directly to those skills and competencies that promote and support personalisation of individuals' needs and preferences. Personalisation and choice in social care is fairly well established through personal budgets and personal care planning, especially following publication of White Papers 'Independence, wellbeing and choice' [11] and 'Our health, our care, our say' [12]. Since 2005, the development of models of social care has focussed on personalisation, independence and choice; the targets set within 'Our health, our care, our say' are those against which social care (both commissioning and provision) is assessed by the regulators.

This competency requires that the practitioner utilises skills both in broader decision-making forums (influencing decision making for commissioning and service planning) and to support and enable decision making at an individual level either through the provision of information and support or through identification of appropriate support structures to enable decision making. The case managers must be able to negotiate with patients and carers the level of representation they will carry out on their behalf, and therefore it is essential that any actions/representations they make are seen as legitimate by service users and others. To ensure the ongoing effectiveness of representation the parameters in which this is delivered must be clear. These parameters must be reviewed regularly to ensure that the service user or carer is still comfortable with the arrangements and that the arrangement is delivering against expectations. This process of review will ensure that any amendments requested or required are recorded and delivered.

Competency B6

This competency supports the delivery of actual outcomes required from B5. The case manager procures effective services and care by representing patient and carer needs in a variety of forums. To procure or commission service the case manager should be able to effectively assess needs, identify how the needs can be met, plan the delivery of the care, if appropriate implement the care and then evaluate how effective the care is, making changes to care plans as required.

Commissioning or procurement requires that the commissioner has an accurate understanding of the services required by patients and their carers. The case manager must then be able to review service providers to identify if there is a provider who can meet the needs locally and if not may need to commission from elsewhere. An ability to understand and define clearly the needs should enable the professional to draw up a clear set of aims and objectives for the care that are measurable, as measures will be required to ensure delivery is in line with specification. The professional must also ensure that the care delivery is safe and effective and of course provided legally.

Once a provider has been identified the procurement process must take place in line with appropriate local and national guidance; many areas use preferred provider models to ensure the safety of this process. The personalisation agenda and extended implementation of personalised budgets to the NHS may complicate this process as patients and carers may wish to commission care themselves from agencies that are not part of this process. They may wish to access services provided from friends and family. This is currently allowed under the social care personal budgeting arrangements, but it is unclear whether the NHS plans will allow this.

The case manager in partnership with the user of care will need to ensure that the provider has the ability to provide the care that is being commissioned. The negotiation of contracts with providers may also form a key skill set for the case manager, the need to ensure value for money in contracts is key in ensuring that public resources are spent appropriately, the requirement for value for money processes is very clear within health and social care [13]. Once care is being delivered then the case managers must use their evaluation skills to monitor effectiveness of care provision; the evaluation must be robust and recorded clearly. Any changes required to improve care delivery must be clearly outlined to enable providers to improve quality, outcomes and cost effectiveness of services. These reviews should be utilised and shared to enable improvements in future contracts.

Competency B7

This competency domain relates directly to skills required in a case manager to ensure the appropriate management of physical resources. The skills in this domain are those that ensure that the professional is mindful of and realistic of resources implications when planning and accessing care. The focus of this area of skill is to ensure that resources are appropriately utilised and managed. Resources are finite and it is necessary to ensure all physical resources (staff, equipment, etc.) are used efficiently. It is expected that a case manager will not just identify for people the resources they need but also ensure that the resources requested are relevant and will deliver appropriate benefits. A resource must have an outcome or benefit that is identified through measurement or evaluation. Being the lead person within a service in relation to resources management, case managers must develop team members and others to understand the importance of effective resource management.

Competency B8

This competency domain relates to the protection of vulnerable people, via this area of competency is delivered the skills within a practitioner that identify and manage any potential vulnerability. The practitioner, to be effective and ensure patient safety, must be able to work with all appropriate individuals to identify situations and events that can result in abuse and danger. The case manager must develop a positive and sensitive relationship that the patient can trust to enable sharing of difficult information. The case manager must be able to identify vulnerability and utilise appropriate processes to protect that person through reporting and managing the process. The area of protection of vulnerable adults is as complex and difficult to manage as safeguarding that of children and guidance exists in all areas to manage any potential issues. These processes and procedures should be followed, as not to do so is to place an already vulnerable person at greater risk.

The case manager being a leader within a service or team should be fully cognisant of vulnerable adult procedures and should be able to act as a role model in this area for team members and other colleagues. The case manager may well need to support staff to whom issues are reported and therefore the case manager should be fully aware of the support processes that are available in the system for staff in this situation.

Identifying high-risk patients, promoting health and preventing ill health

Competency domain G

This competency is aimed at ensuring that the practitioner (usually in this case a community matron) can identify an appropriate caseload of patients who could be defined as high intensity users. The outcomes for these patients would be appropriate health management including prevention of deterioration and promotion of improved health behaviours. To case manage in this context means that the vulnerable high-risk people are identified and provided with proactive and co-ordinated management. These people are usually those who suffer multiple diseases and have highly complex medication and disease interdependencies. The health needs of this patient group is normally difficult because of the multiplicity of practitioners involved in their care; this is the very situation in which co-ordination, or care orchestration as defined in the Evercare model, is most successful.

The key to managing these patients is to identify them effectively. There are a number tools and processes to do this, which have been discussed elsewhere in this text, such as the PAAR tool [14]. The ability to identify appropriate patients for proactive case management is seen as absolutely essential to the level of efficacy of the model of care [15,16]; those case management models that have been able to identify people at risk have managed them well. There remains no real agreement across the NHS on the most effective way of identifying this high-risk group and in most areas a mix of models have been used.

Competency G1

This area of competency relates to the abilities the practitioner must hold to identify, access, structure, analyse, accept, reject and utilise data appropriately. The practitioner must also be able to discuss with the suppliers of information its quality and validity. This process may require use of specialist software and access to specialists in the field of data management. The practitioner should develop the practical skills of literature searching to enable similar pieces of work to be accessed, allowing critical appraisal of the interpretations the practitioner has made alongside the interpretations made by others. The practitioner should also develop the skills to review partial and full data when presented and produce a report or summary of the key issues and findings from analysis and interpretation. The practitioner must work effectively in partnership across sectors and agencies who hold information, understanding the services and priorities of other agencies and how working together can enable delivery of priorities across sectors and organisations. The ability of the practitioner to utilise data systems in public health and other agencies will assist them in the development of an understanding of health profiles and health needs. Skills in this area will enable the practitioner to define and plan to meet local health need and to identify an appropriate caseload of high-risk people which then allows them to be offered appropriate management.

Competency G2

This competency describes the skills and knowledge required in a practitioner to communicate information in relation to health and well-being and the ability to communicate information on those issues that have an adverse impact on health and well-being. Skills within this competency area relate directly to prevention of ill health, protection of health and promotion of self-care.

The practitioner must be able to work in partnership with individuals and group to identify the need for, and develop and disseminate information/ communications in relation to health. The communication must balance the information to be delivered (complexity and nature), outlining the key issues to be understood, and offer options for action and support the audience to make an appropriate decision if it is to be effective. The processes and styles utilised to disseminate information must be appropriate to the nature of the information and the audience, it should therefore be targeted (appropriate to) to its audience. The effectiveness of all communications must be tested; therefore, the practitioner should respond constructively to feedback on communication and make appropriate improvements to ensure efficacy of communication. The ability to identify and share information in an effective and appropriate way requires the practitioner to understand not only the data and the local profile of the area but also all appropriate legislation, guidelines for practice and local service outlines and standards.

For patients and carers this competency provides the support and knowledge that enables an understanding of their health status and its context, the opportunities to change health behaviours and increase confidence and abilities with self-care or management. Patients and carers should through the effective use of this competency by the practitioner be increasingly more in control of their own destiny, which when we review self-care and effectiveness of case management later in this chapter will be seen as one of the most highly valued outcomes of effective case management services.

Competency G3

The ability of a practitioner (case manager) to define the health and well-being needs of their caseload is obviously a key skill for the delivery of the promotion of self-care and the planning and provision of appropriate management for the caseload. The case manager must be able to define the needs of both individuals and the full caseload, presenting the information in effective ways to appropriate people (commissioners, planners and colleagues). The ability to explain the possible course of action and the benefits and risks of these options for care delivery is essential. The information the practitioner collects should be used effectively to prioritise care delivery (both the amount and the time required for delivery). Within this competency area, as with G2, there is a need for the practitioner to be able to balance the complexity of much of the data that will be used and the tensions between organisations and individuals regarding the interpretation and utilisation of data. The practitioner should effectively communicate between differing views, enabling management of any conflicts.

Competency G4

This area of competence requires the practitioner to hold the skills to effectively communicate directly with individuals, groups and communities with regard to the promotion of health and well-being. The practitioner should understand the social constructs of health and how these affect perceptions of health in the population.

The practitioner must be able to effectively define the data and information required to describe health and health risks in relation to the caseload. The ability of individuals, groups or communities to act in an appropriate way to improve or maintain their health and well-being is dependent on the information and knowledge they hold. Professionals in case management roles must be able to, through the provision of information, in appropriate ways, support people to make decisions on health behaviours. This competency relates directly to building the ability in the population to make informed choices and decisions in relation to health and to facilitating self-care/management. The ability to make an informed decision depends on whether the person holds all relevant information. It is the right of person to make their own choices, even if these are wrong choices in the view of professionals. The professional must acknowledge this right and utilise appropriate processes to support and enable correct decisions through the provision of information that a person can use effectively in decision making.

Competency G5

This competency relates to the need for practitioners to ensure health and well-being of their defined caseload through partnership working to reduce health risks and promote health. This area of competence provides the skills required to ensure that exposure to health risks (infection, falls, etc.) is identified and risks mitigated. The case manager must be able to identify individuals whose health and well-being may be at risk. The recognition of risks will enable the practitioner to work with both individuals and other caring professionals to mitigate the risk identified. There are a number of specific areas in which outcomes for patients can be improved using the skills within this competency, such as prevention of infection (advice to care homes on barrier techniques), health promotion (through encouragement and facilitation of vaccination) and improved health outcomes through promotion of self-management (with patients or carers). The practitioner must be able to identify the issues and how these can be managed but they must also be able to share this knowledge effectively and support those involved (staff, patients and carers) to maintain the activities agreed, through regular review and encouragement.

Competency G6

This competency is directly related to the need for practitioners to work in partnership, through influence and negotiation, with communities to improve and maintain their health and well-being. The practitioner working effectively with this competency should be able to support the reduction of health inequalities as required in the operational plan [17]. The effective practitioner should be able to define information for local communities in relation to their health status. The ability to present this information together with options for the community to maintain or improve their health and well-being in an appropriate way and to facilitate the community in its decision making is a fundamental process to the delivery of the wider health improvement strategies in the NHS. Working with communities to assist them to identify and manage their own issues is an effective process for building self-confidence and engagement in health and other community issues. The practitioner must measure the effectiveness of programmes developed for communities through feedback and review, and must use the evaluation/review information to improve effectiveness of processes they utilise. The success of the partnerships between health, local authority and other agencies in developing a sense of belonging to their local communities and engagement in local governance is being assessed through the Comprehensive Area Assessment Framework for Assessment Audit Commission [18].

Interagency and partnership working

Competency I1

The ability to achieve the 'best possible outcomes' for the individual [1] is the main deliverable within this competency area. The outcomes for patients within this competency can be described as promotion and maximisation of participation and independence, prevention of risk and protection from harm. The practitioner must be able to influence the design of services, through planning and procedure development, to ensure these are delivered in a way that enables good outcomes and supports and encourages patients and carers to provide feedback (including making recommendations) on services if they are not doing so. Through the use of this feedback, the practitioner can communicate with service planners and others to improve the delivery of services.

The practitioner should be able to work with and support patient and their carers to recognise risks of abuse and report these safely, making sure that these reports or issues identified are managed appropriately. To enable the safety of service users, it is essential that the practitioner is aware of and work at all times in line with local policies and procedures. Another key area managed within this competency is that of medication safety; within the NHS there are clear requirements, both legislative and professional guidance, in relation to medication safety. All NHS organisations have clear policies in relation to medicines management and medicines safety. Nursing and Midwifery Council has clear guidance in relation to the requirements of good practice in relation to the administration of medication [19] and NICE has recently produced a clinical guideline in relation to Medicines adherence [20]. Both of these documents outline the responsibilities of the professional in relation to the safety of medication and supporting patients in adherence. One of the highest areas of risk for patients, particularly those with complex long-term conditions, is the complexity of their medication regimes, and the likelihood of noncompliance with medication has been identified as having a major impact on successful outcomes for these patients.

Case study

The following case study outline is provided to describe in practice the use of the competencies outlined within this chapter.

Nurse A is a community matron with a caseload of patients with complex needs within a large city in the northwest, the patients are registered with a number of local general practices and approximately half of the caseload are nursing home residents. The supporting team consists of access to a multidisciplinary therapy team, an intermediate care team, general community nursing and other social care services.

Caseload profiling

In line with the requirement of domains G and I the community matron has since her appointment identified the caseload as outlined earlier. Some patients have been referred by medical and other colleagues, but initially the community matron worked with the public health team, commissioning colleagues (admission data) and practices themselves to identify potential high intensity users who could benefit from proactive management. Initially many of the patients were resident in nursing or care homes and this led to a discussion of the service needs for these patients. It was identified that many of patients who had frequent admissions had urological problems (retention, indwelling catheters or recurrent urinary tract infections). After identifying these issues it was decided that a programme of training for nursing and residential home staff in relation to fluid intake, toileting and catheter care including catheterisation would be beneficial. The programme was developed and delivered using appropriate specialists in the three largest residential and nursing homes that had been identified via admission data. The staff were also provided with access to an out of hours advisory service, and the out of hours community nursing team was developed to allow them to provide support as required. The outcome of these support processes was very positive with a reduction of admissions in all three venues. The programme was then further developed for all residential and nursing homes locally.

Patient B is aged 89 and is resident within a nursing home where he has lived for some 5 years. He has a diagnosis of chronic obstructive pulmonary disease (COPD) and mild heart failure. Prior to his admission to the caseload he unfortunately had eight emergency admissions, periods of between 5 and 21 days as an inpatient. On admission to the caseload a full history was defined using patient's own knowledge, general practitioner records (clinical system), nursing home notes and finally access to hospital records. It was clear from this review that a number of differences in understanding existed in relation to Mr B's condition with some confusion regarding medication. The medication confusion in the main was because of delays in communication of medication reviews and changes instigated during hospital admissions and outpatient appointments/follow-ups. Mr B himself was also very confused regarding his medication because of frequent admissions each of which led to some form of medication change. The delays in communication had caused an ongoing issue in relation to appropriate medication changes never being fully implemented effectively.

It was also clear from discussions with nursing home staff and the records that the staff did not fully understand the medical issues Mr B had and were unsure about how he should/could be managed to maintain him in the nursing home despite the fact that he wished for this and they were willing to do so. It was also clear that Mr B was becoming more and more dependent on care because of loss of mobility and lack of confidence following multiple admissions. His loss of mobility was identified as also causing Mr B to have an increased risk of falls and a full falls assessment was completed.

A care plan was developed for Mr B that included a clear description of his medication administration as agreed by his medical team and a clear plan for his long-term care that included physiotherapy support for breathing, falls prevention and mobility. A plan for any exacerbation of his respiratory disease was agreed with the staff, his general practitioner and the patient himself. To support this plan, staff within the nursing home were supported to develop an understanding of the condition, how it progresses and how deteriorations happen to Mr B and what can be done quickly to manage these in line with national guidelines [21,22]. The staff were also given a direct contact number for the service to enable support to be given if required, and a frequent visiting plan was implemented in the short term while Mr B and the staff built their confidence. On three occasions the practitioner was contacted by the staff when Mr B complained of increased breathlessness or cough. On these occasions appropriate action was taken to maintain Mr B within the nursing home and an admission was prevented.

Mr B was also supported to take part in more social interactions much of which he had stopped doing because of lack of confidence and his ongoing concerns regarding his health. The assessment and development of the plan of care was recorded formally to ensure effective communication, continuity of care and safety. The plan also included regular reviews and evaluation of the plan to ensure effectiveness and allow further development if required.

The community matron in this case used very effectively the competencies in domain B by completing a holistic assessment that enabled the development of a care plan based on Mr B's clinical needs and his preference for care. The practitioner used other appropriate services and professionals to improve the health of the patient and to encourage an increased level of independence and social interaction. The practitioner provided development for the nursing home staff through provision of a bespoke training programme (domain G) in relation to COPD, which not only improved care for Mr B but also improved the staff capability to manage the disease in other patients. The safety of the patient was ensured through the robust recognition of risk (falls and medication issues) and an action plan to mitigate the risks (domain I). Finally the practitioner used effective record-keeping skills to ensure the patient was appropriately managed and through the planning of his care reduced the need for emergency admissions.

Mrs C is 76 years old and has diabetes (noninsulin dependent) and heart disease (history of angina for 4 years). For a year she has lived alone following the death of her husband, to whom she had been married for 50 years, and who had been her main support and while she has children (three) none of them live locally. During the previous year Mrs C has had six admissions with episodes of angina. Most of these admissions required less than three days as an inpatient and no abnormal findings had been evident. The cardiology consultant felt that Mrs C was suffering from anxiety following her bereavement. Mrs C was also a nonattendee at chronic disease reviews in the practice despite a number of contacts by the practice staff. Mrs C was referred by her general practitioner to the community matron following the sixth admission.

The community matron arranged to visit Mrs C and prior to the visit reviewed all the clinical records within the general practice. This provided the practitioner with an overview of Mrs C's medical history and an understanding of the level of support that she had received from her husband. At the first visit the practitioner discussed in some detail with Mrs C her health and what had been happening over the previous year, including the admissions and what led to these. Although Mrs C understood her condition fairly well, it became clear that she had been very dependent on her husband who had taken her to see her general practitioner and practice nurse regularly, had ensured concordance with medication and had provided her with support and reassurance. All of these supporting structures had been lost and this did appear to have had a detrimental effect on her ability to cope.

The community matron was able to in partnership with Mrs C develop a plan for her care that included:

- Referral to bereavement support
- Medication advice (dispensing aid)
- Diabetes education support specialist team [23–25]
- Arrangement of appropriate screening (foot and retinal) [23–25]
- Development of coping strategies for anxiety
- Arrangement of support from a social carer (short term)
- Completion of chronic disease reviews to identify any problems

- *Referral to local older peoples group (social)*
- *Regular reviews and evaluation of plans*

These support and care processes gradually improved Mrs C's condition. She was able to understand her medication and to comply with the regime; she was reassured regarding her condition by the full assessment and support by the bereavement group. The development of coping strategies for anxiety reduced significantly any episodes of angina.

The practitioner used domains B, G and I effectively in Mrs C's care through full assessment, reduction of risks and provision of information.

Mrs D was identified as a potential high intensity user during the caseload development stage. She is aged 76 and lives in sheltered accommodation with her husband aged 78. Mrs D had been admitted as an emergency eight times in the previous 6 months each time following a fall. Mrs D suffers from rheumatoid arthritis, diabetes, hypertension and atrial fibrillation. Mrs D is receiving ten different medications including Warfarin.

At the initial assessment it is clear that both Mrs D and her husband have a high level of understanding of her diseases and medication, but Mrs D is becoming unsteady and immobile and because of this is at a high risk of falls. It is also clear from the assessment that she is suffering from urinary frequency that is causing problems, her frequent falls have occurred during her attempts to get quickly to the toilet. It is also very clear that Mrs D's increased immobility is causing problems for Mr D who is becoming less able to offer support or lift her when required. Another key issue identified is the difficulties in relation to attendance at regular anticoagulation reviews that have caused major anxiety to the couple because of mobility and falls issues. Both the carer and the patient are anxious to maintain a level of independence and to remain together, but both are anxious regarding the future and this is causing friction between them.

The practitioner using her knowledge and skills is able to develop a plan of care to support both the patient and the carer through:

- *Therapy assessment regarding mobility, moving and handling and falls prevention including equipment and environment.*
- *Review of medication to ensure all is required*
- *Arrangement of short-term home anticoagulation reviews*
- *Referral to support via social care system for general care (bathing, etc.)*
- *Support and contact advice for emergencies and general support.*
- *Referral of carer to local carer support service*
- *Regular reviews and evaluation of condition to effectiveness of plan*

The care plan and interventions allowed a marked improvement in the couple's lives, Mrs D was able to build her confidence and improve her mobility, and Mr D was able to continue caring for his wife. Mrs D reported feeling better, she did not require any further admissions because of falls and was able to manage much better. Mrs D was able to take her medication appropriately and safely with regular and appropriate review particularly in relation to her anticoagulant therapy. The practitioner utilised competencies in domain B and G in a highly effective way for this couple.

Conclusion

Delivery of the skills and knowledge required for the competencies described in this chapter provide for patients and their carers practitioners highly effective care. The competencies enable positive outcomes in the care delivered; the role of case manager is to make a positive impact on the care of patients with chronic long-term conditions, patients and carers who live with highly complex health needs. The competencies in domains B, G and I are not used in isolation from other competencies but this chapter provides some detail in relation to the impact the competencies discussed can have on patients and carers and the experience of care they receive.

References

1. Department of Health (2006). *Caring for People with Long Term Conditions: An Education Framework for Community Matrons and Case Managers.* http://www.dh.gov.uk/prod_consum_dh/groups/dh_digitalassets/@dh/@en/documents/digitalasset/dh_4118102.pdf (accessed on October 2009).
2. UnitedHealth Europe (2005). *Assessment of Evercare Programme in England 2003–2004.* http://www.dh.gov.uk/prod_consum_dh/groups/dh_digitalassets/@dh/@en/documents/digitalasset/dh_4114224.pdf (accessed on October 2009).
3. Department of Health (2009). *Reference Guide to Consent to Examination or Treatment.* http://www.dh.gov.uk/prod_consum_dh/groups/dh_digitalassets/documents/digitalasset/dh_103653.pdf (accessed on October 2009).
4. House of Lords House of Commons (2007). *The Human Rights of Older People in Healthcare Eighteenth Report of Session 2006-07 Joint Committee of Human Rights.* http://www.publications.parliament.uk/pa/jt200607/jtselect/jtrights/156/15602.htm
5. Department of Health (2009). *NHS Constitution.* http://www.dh.gov.uk/prod_consum_dh/groups/dh_digitalassets/documents/digitalasset/dh_093442.pdf (accessed on October 2009).
6. Help the Aged & Picker Institute (2008). *Measuring Dignity in Care for Older People: A research Report for Help the Aged.* http://policy.helptheaged.org.uk/NR/rdonlyres/EFD769F8-930A-412E-B079-FD058EE6AA69/0/on_our_own_terms_021208.pdf
7. Department of Health (2008). *High Quality Care for All NHS Next Stage Review. Final Report.* http://www.dh.gov.uk/prod_consum_dh/groups/dh_digitalassets/@dh/@en/documents/digitalasset/dh_085828.pdf (accessed on October 2009).
8. Goodrich J and Cornwell J (2008). *Seeing the Person in the Patient. The Point of Care Review Paper.* King's Fund. http://www.kingsfund.org.uk/applications/site_search/?term=Seeing+the+person+in+the+patient&searchreferer_id=2&submit.x=36&submit.y=8 (accessed on October 2009).

9. Department of Health (2006). *Records Management NHS Code of Conduct Part 1.* http://www.dh.gov.uk/prod_consum_dh/groups/dh_digitalassets/@dh/@en/documents/digitalasset/dh_4133196.pdf (accessed on October 2009).

10. Department of Health (2009). *Records Management NHS Code of Conduct Part 2.* http://www.dh.gov.uk/prod_consum_dh/groups/dh_digitalassets/documents/digitalasset/dh_093024.pdf (accessed on October 2009).

11. Secretary of State for Health (March 2005). *Independence, Well-being and Choice: Our Vision for the future of Social Care for Adults in England.* http://www.dh.gov.uk/prod_consum_dh/groups/dh_digitalassets/@dh/@en/documents/digitalasset/dh_4106478.pdf (accessed on October 2009).

12. Department of Health (2006). *Our Health, Our Care, Our Say: A New Direction for Community Services.* http://www.dh.gov.uk/prod_consum_dh/groups/dh_digitalassets/@dh/@en/documents/digitalasset/dh_4127459.pdf (accessed on October 2009).

13. Audit Commission (2009). *Use of Resources Framework: Overall Approach and Key Lines of Enquiry.* May 2008 updated February 2009. http://www.audit-commission.gov.uk/localgov/audit/UoR/Pages/uor200809.aspx (accessed on October 2009).

14. King's Fund, NYU Centre for Health and Public Services (2006). *Combined Predictive Model Executive Summary of Interim Results Health Dialog.* http://www.kingsfund.org.uk/applications/site_search/?term=Combined+Predictive+Model+Executive+Summary+of+Interim+Results+&oldterm=Seeing+the+person+in+the+patient&old_term=Seeing+the+person+in+the+patient&old_instance_id=180516&submit.x=28&submit.y=14 (accessed on October 2009).

15. Department of Health (2005). *Supporting People with Long Term Conditions: An NHS and Social Model to Support Local Innovation and Integration.* http://www.dh.gov.uk/prod_consum_dh/groups/dh_digitalassets/@dh/@en/documents/digitalasset/dh_4122574.pdf (accessed on October 2009).

16. Essex Strategic Health Authority (December 2004). Strategic Framework for Case management of Long Term Conditions. http://www.dhsspsni.gov.uk/case_management.pdf

17. Department of Health (2008). *High Quality Care for All: The Operating Framework for the NHS in England 2009/10.* http://www.dh.gov.uk/prod_consum_dh/groups/dh_digitalassets/@dh/@en/documents/digitalasset/dh_091446.pdf (accessed on October 2009).

18. Audit Commission (2009). *Comprehensive Area Assessment Framework for Assessment.* http://www.audit-commission.gov.uk/SiteCollectionDocuments/MethodologyAndTools/Guidance/caaframework10feb09REP.pdf (accessed on October 2009).

19. Nursing & Midwifery Council (2008).*Standards for the Administration of Medicines.* http://www.nmc-uk.org/aDisplayDocument.aspx?DocumentID=6228 (accessed on October 2009).

20. NICE (2009). *Medicines Adherence: Involving Patients in Decision about Prescribing Medicines and Supporting Adherence.* NICE Clinical Guidelines 76. http://guidance.nice.org.uk/CG76 (accessed on October 2009).

21. NationalCollaboratingCentreforChronicConditions(2004).*ChronicObstructivePulmonary Disease. National Guidelines on the Management of Chronic Obstructive Pulmonary Disease in Adults in Primary and Secondary Care.* http://guidance.nice.org.uk/CG12 (accessed on October 2009).

22. Healthcare Commission (2006). Clearing the Air: A National Study of Chronic Obstructive Pulmonary Disease. http://www.cqc.org.uk/_db/_documents/COPD_report1_200607272728.pdf

23. Department of Health (2003). *National Service Framework for Diabetes*. http://www. dh.gov.uk/prod_consum_dh/groups/dh_digitalassets/@dh/@en/documents/ digitalasset/dh_4058938.pdf (accessed on October 2009).
24. Department of Health (2006). *Turning the Corner: Improving Diabetes Care*. Report from Dr Sue Roberts National Clinical Director for Diabetes. http://www.dh.gov.uk/ prod_consum_dh/groups/dh_digitalassets/@dh/@en/documents/digitalasset/ dh_4136011.pdf (accessed on October 2009).
25. Diabetes UK (2007). Diabetes: State of the Nations 2006. Progress Made in Delivering the National Diabetes Frameworks. A Report from Diabetes UK. http://www.diabetes. org.uk/documents/reports/sotn2006_full.pdf

Chapter 5
Outcomes for Patients – Advanced Nursing Practice

Introduction

The management and support to patients with long-term conditions, who need complex care, and their carers, requires a high level of knowledge and skills within practitioners. The delivery of the services for these complex patients requires practitioners to function in a complex care environment and the development of case management competency domains to underpin educational frameworks for the development of the practitioners [1]. The domains reviewed in this chapter are related to assessment and planning of services for an individual, facilitation and support of teams through excellent leadership practice, skills that enable support to individuals undergoing transition and facilitation and delivery of learning and education. These competencies would be relevant in all case management roles, though those relating to physical examination may be specific to nursing and allied health professional groups. The chapter outlines in some detail the competency definitions linked to possible and expected outcomes. The chapter also includes a case study to highlight some of the outcomes that can and have been delivered to patients and their carers by case management processes. The domains that will be reviewed are A, C, F and H.

Advanced clinical nursing practice

Competency A1

This competency outlines the requirement on the case manager to gather information relating to an individual to perform an effective assessment. The information would be in the form of a full health, medical and social history and would include main problems and a full system assessment (cardiac, respiratory, neurological, vascular, endocrine, etc.). The skills used would allow all appropriate information to be collected from patients and carers (professional and non professional). The practitioner should be clear in their explanations to patients and carers regarding their role and the reason for the request for information. To access this information the practitioner will need to use effective communication skills and must be mindful of the private and sometimes sensitive nature of some of the information they will be collecting. It is essential that the practitioner uses safe and effective systems to store information [2,3] and that the information stored is accurate and recorded in a systematic and logical manner, treating this at all times as confidential [4]. The practitioner must also be mindful of the need to obtain informed consent to share information with other agencies and professionals [5]. To ensure access to all information the practitioner will need to use appropriate questioning techniques to explore and clarify information provided. The practitioner will need to be mindful of the broader communication needs of those who require interpretation or other communication support, as this will affect the success of communication with these patient groups.

The practitioner requires a broad understanding of clinical systems (body systems) and the normal ranges and abnormal ranges to allow them to interpret their findings effectively. The practitioner needs to understand the time frames in which information needs to be accessed (presenting symptoms, recent history) and how these time frames will affect the usefulness of the information. The practitioner needs to be a highly experienced communicator and be able to use this experience to manage communication difficulties with patients and carers. The practitioner also needs to understand the impact of an individual's belief system on the information they may or may not provide and the need to respect these beliefs.

The full assessment of an individual by using these skills is the only effective and safe way of determining the needs of a patient and their carers; insufficient or inaccurate information is highly dangerous and can lead to poor outcomes for patients. Another key skill is the ability to carry out an assessment of the mental health status of an individual by using appropriate assessment tools. A highly skilled practitioner is required to complete this full assessment which includes a physical or clinical examination or mental health assessment, but for those patients with chronic medical conditions the practitioner should be able to carry out a full physical examination as the medical condition must be assessed and risk rated to allow care planning to be defined.

Competency A2

This competency relates to the skills and knowledge held by the practitioner in relation to assessment of functional capabilities; the type of tests would include mobility, function, cognition and perception. For an effective outcome the assessments must be completed in a safe environment and the patient must be fit enough to take part. The practitioner must explain clearly the function of the assessment, including who the information from the assessment may be shared with once completed, and ensure the patient has consented to the process. The process of the assessment must define the capability of the patient, should be recorded clearly and accurately and should be appropriate and thorough. Once the assessment and evaluation is completed the outcome will be used to influence and plan the care for the individual. The findings of the assessment may also be used as part of the referral information to another agency, specialist or professional to access care for the patient.

Effective use of this competency will ensure that a patient is assessed effectively and safely, and that the assessment identifies any risk issues for the patient and carers. The practitioner completing the assessment will through their knowledge of normal function, contraindications and progress of conditions be able to assess deviations in function and develop plans to manage the impact or reduce the deviation in line with national guidance and legislation. The outcomes of this competency for patients and carers relate directly to the promotion and maintenance of independence and safety for patients and their carers.

Competency A3

A practitioner who effectively delivers this competency is able to investigate and diagnose an individual who is unwell. This competency requires that the practitioner can utilise their knowledge and skills to clinically examine a patient who is unwell. The practitioner must be able to utilise clinical examination and investigation skills required to assess a clinical condition. The skills used may require auscultation, percussion, palpation, vocal resonance and functional examination [6]. The practitioner must be able to very quickly identify the ability of the individual to understand their condition and make appropriate decisions.

The practitioner must be able to assess the condition of the patient medically by utilising knowledge of the medical condition, including how it progresses. Using this knowledge the practitioner can then decide on the management approach for the patient. It is essential for the safety of the patient that the practitioner can recognise how serious the condition is and assess the risk to the patient, identifying when managing the condition is outside their level of competence or requires acute medical intervention. The assessment may require initiation and interpretation of investigations such as x-ray or blood chemistry. The practitioner must be able to identify abnormal results and ensure appropriate action is taken either by themselves or by referral to an appropriate practitioner.

It is essential that the practitioner uses a systematic and logical approach to assessment, and that the examination and all findings are accurately recorded alongside actions taken or planned. Patients being proactively managed through case management will present with exacerbations of their conditions; they may also present with new conditions that require initial and ongoing management. It is essential that a practitioner can recognise and differentiate between existing and deteriorating conditions and new issues to ensure the safe and effective management of the patient.

The effectiveness of case managers in this domain is normally evident through early recognition and management of changes in conditions, which can be existing or new. Practitioners who have these skills are able to manage patients proactively and it is clear from the evaluations of case management [7] that these patients report 'feeling better' in general terms and their use of emergency services are reduced.

Competency A4

This competency relates to the development, implementation, monitoring and evaluation of care plans. The development of a care plan/programme depends on thorough assessment and complete understanding of the history, condition and expectations of a patient and their carers. The care plan must provide a clear process by which the needs of patient and their carers are to be met. It must be developed in partnership with the patient and their carer and must be realistic in expectation. The development of the plan is the second stage in case management. It requires that the case manager agrees the key problems with the patient and their carer, and they agree with the plan for management. The plan must clearly define what the expected outcome is for the patient and carer. The plan may include referral to other agencies and multiagency service provision. Any care intervention must be delivered in an appropriate environment to ensure the safety of the patient.

The consent of the patient is essential for all interventions [5], and as some patients may have difficulties in relation to capacity to give consent, the practitioner must be mindful of the legal requirements for these patients [8]. The patient must, if appropriate, receive a clear explanation of all interventions to ensure they are aware of risks and benefits. This will enable them to make an informed decision. The practitioner should effectively engage the patient and their carer in any decision regarding their care. To ensure this the practitioner should provide to patients and carers in an understandable way information on the effectiveness of any specific intervention or management approach.

To ensure that the monitoring and evaluation of care plan and process is carried out effectively, it is essential that the patient and carer are involved in the process. This requires that the practitioner has excellent communication and engagement skills that facilitate and encourage this involvement. The ability of patients and carers to comment on the success or failure of a plan of care must be developed as it is fundamental to the success of case management that patients and carers own the process of care and are fully engaged in it. This engagement is part of the development of self-care and management skills for them. All said and done, it is their care and therefore they should be able to express their views on its efficacy. While historically it is not necessarily routine for patients to always voice their views on care, the practitioner may need to spend time with the patient and carer outlining the reason for the process. The NHS has for many years struggled to evidence that it listens to patient's comments; although the situation has improved slightly in recent years [9], it may require extra effort to make involvement in evaluation of care routine in the NHS. Social care has used service user and carer involvement in reviews of care packages for a number of years in a highly effective way [10] and the NHS has much to learn from this process. The practitioner must be able to recognise when an external issue is affecting the outcome of a care programme and to make appropriate arrangements to reduce the negative impact if possible. The ability of the practitioner to use care planning and evaluation to develop reports and information that ensures efficient admission and discharge processes and prevents delays is also fundamental to this skills area.

This competency delivers outcomes in relation to safe and effective care planning and delivery for patients and their carers. It is the area in which implementation of care is set. If the assessment carried out is robust and the care planned is appropriate, and the delivery is effective and efficient, then the planned or expected outcomes for patients and carers must be delivered. To ensure the outcomes are delivered, monitoring and evaluation is the key. Patients expect that the planned care will be delivered, but sometimes the delivery of care is completed by an external agency and it may not be delivered as planned. Ongoing monitoring and regular evaluation will enable problems, if they occur, to be identified and managed quickly, which probably will prevent or reduce any negative impacts on the patient or their carer.

Competency A5

This competency relates to the assessment of needs in those patients who are reaching the end-of-life stage of their condition. Many of the current long-term conditions will eventually progress to an end stage. This end stage with most of these diseases is now long term, but eventually the time will come when management of the disease becomes palliation (management of symptoms). The ability to support the individual to make an informed and appropriate decision on their preferences for end-of-life care is highly important in the case management roles. The case manager should be able to assess the condition of the patient and identify when the end-of-life stage is being reached, which will be done in partnership with specialist services. The patient's preferences for care should be clearly defined to enable choice and ensure that they are treated with the dignity and respect they deserve [11,12].

End-of-life care requires that all involved have been part of the decision and planning. An effective assessment of the condition including regular reviews and evaluation is also essential to ensure that changes in the condition are identified early as this allows good management of symptoms and ensures that the patient is kept comfortable. The need to ensure that the individual's preferences and views are at the centre of all care is a fundamental tenant of this type of care and ensures that their human rights are protected [13]. The ability to work in partnership with other agencies to provide care services to patients at the end of life requires that the practitioner holds an understanding of differing philosophies, principles and code of practice in partner agencies and a thorough knowledge of their policies and procedures. This level of understanding will ensure that appropriate care can be requested and delivered in line with the needs identified and planned.

When care is being delivered, ongoing evaluation of the condition of the patient, the effectiveness of the care plan and the preferences of the patient must continue. Choices and decisions can and do change and the practitioner must recognise as quickly as possible when a situation has changed and care plan needs to be reviewed and updated. All information on assessments, plans and reviews must be recorded in line with national and professional codes of conduct and must be kept in line with guidance on confidentiality and record-keeping.

The ability of a case manager to support a patient and their carer through the end-of-life stage can be very rewarding. To ensure a patient dies with dignity and in peace, in the way in which they chose, with family and friends around them is a highly successful outcome for the patient and carer. It can be upsetting and may cause anxiety for the carer, but with competent care and support these anxieties can be reduced and the experience can be acceptable while still upsetting.

Competency A6

This competency relates to the safe and effective use of medicines. Patients who have long-term conditions are likely to be prescribed a wide range of medicine; in fact, there is evidence that they are likely to be prescribed five or more medications. It is also clear from the evidence that the more medication a patient takes the more problems they will have in relation to compliance issues and poli-pharmacy issues [14]. Prescribed medication accounts for 15% of all health expenditure [15].

The ability to support requires that the practitioner develops a supportive relationship with the individual, which will allow the practitioner to assess the patients understanding of their medication regime, assess the appropriateness of the regime and the level of concordance with it. It is essential that the patient understands what a medicine is for, how and when to take it and what to expect from the medication if we expect them to comply with the regime. Patients who are supported to understand these issues are more likely to make the decision to comply with medicines prescribed to them [15].

The practitioner must at all times work within their level of competency and in line with their appropriate professional codes and national guidelines in relation to medication. The professional should ensure that they identify the current (up-to-date) medication the patient has been prescribed. They should be mindful of the fact that a patient having multiple conditions may be reviewed by a number of practitioners all of whom may prescribe, and this may mean that the actual medication being taken by the patient is different from that recorded in the clinical record in primary care. Any differences in medication must be investigated and appropriate action taken to confirm the medication being prescribed. This action alone may immediately improve the situation for the patient because confusion with medication is a major problem for patients, particularly those who have multiple conditions or frequent admissions. The practitioner must be able to understand and recognise the potential side effects of medication prescribed for a patient, identify the risks of medication prescribed and be cognisant of drug interdependencies at all times, ensuring the safety of the patient through effective and accurate record-keeping.

The outcomes delivered by the practitioner through this competency relate directly to improved health and well-being, safety and concordance with medication regimes. Patients who are supported by a knowledgeable and effective practitioner will be more likely to understand their medication and there will be less confusion regarding their drug regime. Reduction in waste of drugs in the NHS will be a by-product of this competency though it is not the most important.

Competency A7

This competency is aimed at delivery of the skills required for prescribing practice in case management; prescribing (independent or supplementary dependent on professional background) requires that the practitioner can examine and diagnose the patient, make a differential diagnosis and decision on treatment and management through the provision of medicine. To be a prescriber the practitioner must complete an appropriate prescribing programme as outlined by the appropriate professional body. Each professional body has agreed the learning requirements for the programme and all require that the practitioner is able to assess, examine clinically and diagnose prior to prescribing.

Proactively manage complex long-term conditions

Competency C1

This domain represents the competencies required to proactively manage complex long-term conditions and competency C1 relates to the ability of a practitioner to plan, implement, monitor and review individual care plans with individuals who have a long-term condition. To deliver the outcomes expected of this competency, the practitioner must be able to develop effective relationships with individuals and key people. Using these relationships, they should provide information to support decision making regarding care and services that the patient may choose to access and ensure that the patient is in a position to communicate their needs while balancing the rights of the individual against those of the wider community. The practitioner must work in a partnership with patients and carers and with service providers to facilitate patient choice. The practitioner must be able to use their skills to enable conflicts and dilemmas to be managed. One of the skills that patients and carers may need to develop is the ability to challenge, comment and complain when services are not appropriate to their needs and to do so in a way that is fair and does not expose them to any risk of unfair treatment. Older patients may be reluctant to complain or voice concerns and case manager must act at all times to ensure that their voices are heard. This competency also outlines the need to support patients and carers in accessing appropriate external support and advocacy if required, a key requirement if a patient does not have the capacity to act on their own behalf as defined by the advice relating to the Mental Capacity Act [16]. It is expected that the practitioner using this competency effectively will support the patient and carers to ensure that actions and decisions are in line with their human rights as described within the report of the Joint Committee on Human Rights in Healthcare [17] and ensures respect for beliefs, culture and values. The patient outcomes from this competency are likely to be reported in the views on patient and carer experience as this competency is all about delivering care in line with the needs and views of patients themselves and if care is delivered in this way then the experience for patients must be improved.

Competency C2

To enable the delivery of patient-centred care as defined in several policy documents [18,19], the patient and their carers must be involved in the process of developing care plan; the patient must influence and agree the content of plans as without this how can we be sure that the plan developed can meet the needs the patients have. Competency C2 is totally focussed on the abilities required in the practitioner that enable them to assess (identify) the needs patients have and agree how these needs will be met through service delivery and support. The assessment for needs must reflect the patients' understanding of their needs as it is not unusual for an issue that is identified as important by a professional to be viewed by the patient as unimportant and easy to cope with. The professional must assess the individuals' understanding of their condition through a description of their health and review with the individual what the problems and issues may be and what they are capable to self-manage, which must include an understanding of their attitude to self-management (commitment and motivation). Once all information has been gathered and any examination needed has been completed the overall condition will be defined, which must include an understanding of any long-term complication from the diseases the patient may be suffering. The practitioner must then access any risk to the patient, which will be done against agreed guidelines. Delivery of the processes outlined will ensure that the plan of care that is implemented is based on the needs of the patient, which have been clearly defined during the assessment and are understood. This process enables the delivery of a care plan that is based on this knowledge and understanding which the patient has agreed. A patient-centred and agreed plan of care must by definition provide better outcomes for patients and is therefore the best outcome indicator in this competency area.

Competency C3

This competency requires the practitioner to enable individuals with long-term conditions to make informed choices concerning their health and well-being. The ability to deliver this requires further development of the relationship between the patient and the practitioner as a supportive relationship allows the practitioner to use communication skills to encourage the patient to question and challenge information and seek appropriate clarification regarding the plans and processes being used in their care. The practitioner must communicate effectively to ensure that the patient has all the information they need to make choices in relation to their health and well-being and to decide on the most appropriate option for their care. An effective practitioner will also encourage the patient to review the choices they have made to ensure a decision or choice made remains the right one for them and support the patient to access information or advice externally if appropriate to ensure they are properly informed. The ability of patients to make decisions for themselves is important as it allows them to have a sense of ownership of the processes of care, which is often missing for patients with long-term conditions. Ownership and influence on care planning and programmes is felt to improve the level of concordance with care and builds the capacity in the patient to self-care/manage. This process of involvement and ownership in care planning through choice means that the patient can fully understand the interventions and can give informed consent to the intervention. The outcomes in relation to this competency for patients are clearly that of ownership and control; patients report that their experience of care is better when they are involved in processes of planning and can make choices regarding what happens to them.

Competency C4

This competency relates directly to how the practitioner supports a patient to live in a home maintaining independence. To live in their own home the patient must understand their strengths and skills and identify the support they may need to enable them to remain in their own environment. Patients with long-term conditions should understand any risks to themselves that are caused through their condition or the effects of their condition. The assessment of the personal, psychological, physical, financial and social support needs should be clearly defined and the support should be identified and accessed either by the patient themselves or through referral from the practitioner. This competency is all about supporting and enabling the patient to live in their own home safely with the required support, which is about supporting the independence of the patient and promoting self-management/care and of course ownership of their health and the management being provided. Patients who are supported to be independent in this way are more confident of their health and have a greater feeling of control of their lives, which is often the first thing that is lost when a patient becomes ill with a long-term condition.

Competency C5

This competency is focussed on the ability of the practitioner to build partnerships between teams, patients and carers and provides further support to the patient in relation to involvement and control of their care. This competency outlines the importance of not just the involvement of patients in decisions but of the need for the decisions made to be acted upon and the need to ensure in an ongoing way that the patient, carers and care team are all clear and that there are no misunderstandings between the partners. The effectiveness of the partnership with the patient must be evaluated and reviewed as the ongoing delivery of care which meets the needs of the patient relies on the communication between the professional and the patient and carers.

Competency C6

This competency also focusses on partnerships but in relation to maintaining and ensuring the safety of all involved in care. Patients and carers must be kept safe and the professional must operate within the limits of their competency to ensure the safety and effectiveness of care. They must also work with all legal and other frameworks to ensure the safety of staff, patients and carers, which would include security, health and safety. The practitioner is required to use their skill to identify and assess any health safety or security issues and report these, ensuring appropriate actions are taken to reduce and manage the risks. Effective use of this competency ensures the safety of patients and carers and enables care to be delivered safely.

Professional practice and leadership

Competency F1

This competency is all about the provision of clinical leadership, ensuring personal development and professional development of staff. Staff delivering care to patients must be competent; they must have completed all appropriate training they require to deliver treatments and interventions, which would include mandatory training such as safeguarding adults and health and safety. Ensuring staff are appropriately trained and skilled is a leadership function. Leaders in organisations are expected to set the standards in relation to training, which ensure compliance with the Standards for Better Health [20], and all professionals are required by their professional codes to ensure that they are appropriately skilled and trained for any intervention they are delivering, the code for nurses [21] clearly states that a nurse must not undertake any intervention that is outside his/her competence. As a community matron or case manager, the practitioner should support staff and colleagues in identifying gaps in knowledge and skills and in accessing training to meet these needs. The practitioner will also be expected to provide mentorship and tutoring support, including assessment of skills for members of the team. For patients this competency delivers quality and safe care, without appropriate skills and knowledge practitioners cannot deliver safe care.

Competency F2

The ability of staff to provide evidence-based care requires that leaders promote the values and principles that underpin best practice. This competency ensures the delivery of care in line with evidence-based guidelines. Patients and carers rely on practitioners to do the right thing at the right time and to do this effectively requires that practitioner have access to evidence regarding practice and are able to utilise this information, converting it into care delivery. The NHS has a number of processes through which evidence-based guidelines are published to enable the delivery of care in line with good practice, National Service Frameworks, National Institute of Clinical Excellence guidelines and pathways of care. All these guides are produced for the NHS as part of the progress to ensure that all pathways of care and other interventions are based on robust evidence as this is seen as fundamental to the delivery of care which is safe and effective.

Competency F3

This competency supports the requirements within all professional codes that practitioners act at all times within the limits of their competence and authority. Each professional body outlines this expectation within its code of conduct or practice. There can be no debate that it is both reasonable and sensible for the public to expect that practitioners are cognisant of their abilities and competencies so that they do not undertake any intervention or action which is outside these. The practitioner must recognise any gaps in their knowledge and skills and take action to develop the skills, but they must also be able to recognise when an intervention requires delivery by an appropriate specialist and take the required action to refer the patient to the specialist. In this subset there is also an expectation that the practitioner will review for appropriateness the policies and protocols being utilised to deliver care for patients. The nature of health care is such that practice develops and moves on. It is therefore essential to the ongoing delivery of care that pathways and care processes are regularly reviewed for compliance with known good practice.

It is also important for both patient and staff safety that professionals are aware of any area of practice that is outside their authority; for example, prescribing rights are restricted by law to certain professional groups who meet the required criteria. In many ways this competency underpins the safety of patients, each subset provides clarity of expectation on professionals in areas that are understood to directly affect the ability of a practitioner to do their job appropriately.

Competency F4

This subset describes the expectations of a practitioner in relation to leadership to facilitate the development of organisational policy and practice that includes influencing the aims and objectives of the organisation or service. The case management practitioner is a highly skilled practitioner on whom there is an expectation of delivery of improved organisational practice and policy. The practitioner should be involved in ensuring that policy and practice either during initial development or on review are produced and implemented across the organisation. Leadership roles in organisations are essential in helping the organisation or service to maintain a focus on the delivery of its objectives, and leaders must be able to influence and be role model for staff in the organisation or service. The NHS has for many years been focussing on the development of leadership in the organisations through the implementation of a number of leadership programmes [22–24]. All programmes aim to improve the capacity and capability of leaders and specifically in 'Inspiring leaders: leadership for quality', guidance for NHS talent and leadership plans, the Department of Health clearly sets out the need for excellence in leadership to influence the quality, safety and patient experience across all services. The impact on outcomes for patients of this area of competence is obvious in that the skills and knowledge underpin all professional practice and could be seen as responsible for all areas of quality and safety.

Competency F5

This subset defines the skills required in a practitioner to develop, sustain and evaluate collaborative work. The ability to work collaboratively is in many ways the bedrock of case management practice. Unless a practitioner is skilled in this area, delivery of co-ordinated and seamless service to patients will not happen. The practitioner must be able to influence collaboration through identification of both advantages and disadvantages to the organisation, which will include a clear understanding of the purpose of the collaboration and how the aims of collaborating organisations can be delivered through the collaboration.

A modern NHS as defined by the recent Darzi review [25] and the operating framework [26] requires that both commissioners and providers, and therefore practitioners, identify opportunities to develop partnerships and collaborations to enable the delivery of care closer to communities. Services are more and more being commissioned from providers who are not necessarily part of the NHS family, and many services are being delivered through voluntary and nonstatutory providers. Practitioners must therefore have the appropriate skills to build partnerships with a number of agencies. The ability to build partnerships and collaborations will also enable the practitioner to work with agencies to evaluate the effectiveness and appropriateness of services and influence service change if required, which will ensure that services delivered as part of these collaborations are being delivered appropriately and are meeting the needs of patients.

The practitioner must also develop the skills to work in collaboration with communities. A number of policy documents from the Department of Health and reports for organisations such as the King's Fund have outlined the need for the NHS [25,27,28] to change its approach from managing sickness into promoting wellness. This move to engaging the public in their own health focusses on prevention of the preventable diseases and encourages communities to take part in programmes that improve the health of the community as a whole. How the NHS works with partners such as local authorities to deliver their local area agreements and the effectiveness of these partnerships will be assessed via the Comprehensive Area Assessment (CAA) that will be completed each year for each local authority and all its partner agencies [29]. For CAA to be delivered and to make a real difference to the health and well-being of local communities, the partnerships that are responsible for delivering must be effective.

Managing care at the end of life

Competency H1

This competency supports those patients who are going through what is defined as a 'significant life event or transition' such as a diagnosis that has a poor prognosis and the deterioration of a condition or a diagnosis that will negatively affect a person's ability to live independently. Families and carers must also be supported at this time. It is essential that practitioners are able to assess the need for support and provide this or refer as appropriate. It is clear from this subset definition that case management practitioners are expected to influence and encourage the development of services that will support patients and carers at the end of life. Although it may not always be appropriate for the practitioner to provide all the support required, the professional must develop and maintain good relationships with specialist services. If support is being provided by the practitioners own team or linked services, the practitioner should ensure that those delivering the support and care have the appropriate skills and competencies to do so effectively and safely. Staff involved in this type of support processes must be experienced enough to recognise when the needs of the patient or carers become more complex or are outside their skills and abilities. If staff are unable to do this it could expose a patient or carer to an increased level of risk. Practitioners must be able to identify and measure the ability of patient and carers to manage the stress and anxiety during transition. The practitioner should ensure that the patient and carer maintain an appropriate level of control and that the needs in relation to this are reviewed regularly as these may change.

The practitioner may be in a position to influence commissioning and/or service planning and therefore should ensure that opportunities to develop the support services required are not missed. The practitioner should be able to champion the development of procedures and processes to provide support to patients and carers, ensuring that once implemented the processes are regularly reviewed so that they remain effective. Effective support services for patients and carers should be available across the range of transition times, which would include support for managing a changed self view if a patient becomes disabled and preparing for end of life and the bereavement process. The improving outcomes guidelines for palliative care and its supporting evidence [30,31] clearly set the standards for the support that should be available for patients and carers at the end of life. Provision of good support during these difficult periods can deliver a huge impact for patients and carers; it can enable families and their loved ones to make a difficult situation at least tolerable.

Competencies H2 and H3

Though this competency subsets have the same overarching, descriptor H2 relates to supporting the patient during the delivery of the 'bad news' and H3 relates to the support provided in the period after the message is given and how the practitioner supports patients and carers to cope with the change in situation. The practitioner should ensure that the environment is appropriate (privacy) when a patient and their carers are being informed about a poor prognosis and that the follow-up advice and support is made available, such as specialist advice, contact arrangements, follow-up for support and communication with primary care.

Patients and carers have reported terrible experiences when they were given 'bad news', which included being informed in the middle of clinic or ward, with no privacy or follow-up support. After the news is given, the patients and carers should be supported to access any advice or other information that they might need to plan for care in the future. The practitioner must be able to assess the ongoing need for support as the situation may change and the patient may need to be referred for specialist support. The mental health status of patients and carers will need to be regularly assessed to ensure that referral for appropriate support can be made and the support is provided.

The practitioner should have the ability to communicate effectively with patients and carers to enable assessment, planning and implementation of support to meet the patient needs. The practitioner must ensure that information regarding the needs of patients and carers is shared appropriately within confidentiality and information sharing agreements. The support needed for carers and family to prepare for the bereavement process must also be identified and the support accessed through referral or care planning.

Case study 1

Practitioner E is a community matron within a large city, she has been newly appointed to manage a new caseload that consists of patients within a group of nursing homes. The practitioner will link to a team of community practitioners (2 band 5 nurses, 2 support workers band 3), the community-based therapy staff and the community intermediate care team. All the nursing home patients have been identified as having multiple chronic conditions, and a review of activity in relation to emergency admissions has identified that among the patients' resident in the home there appear to be a number who have had frequent emergency admissions over the last 3 months. The nursing staff in the home appear to have poor relationships with the general practices with whom the patients are registered, and there is no obvious history of reviews of the patients' chronic conditions.

The practitioner begins her role by working with the nursing home to review the patients who have been admitted as an emergency in the previous 6 months. This review identified across the 4 homes of 120 beds 35 patients who had been admitted twice or more over the 6-month period. The review also identified that calls to out of hours services were also an issue. The practitioner also gained an understanding of the capacity and capability of the supporting teams to ensure referrals for support were appropriate to the supporting teams' abilities.

The practitioner then commenced a review of all the patients' records, both clinical (GP) and nursing home, using the information to prioritise patients for full clinical assessment. The prioritisation exercise was based on the level of risk to the patient (number of diagnoses, nursing home report on current condition, number of medicines, recent out of hours visits, etc.). Gradually in a planned way the community matron assessed the prioritised patients and from these assessments was able to define a programme of care for each patient that was agreed with the patient if appropriate and with the staff within the nursing home. Each plan of care developed was individualised and contained advice for staff on how to identify early changes in condition and how to access advice to manage the changes or to implement a programme of care to arrest the deterioration. To ensure that the nursing home staff were able to deliver these plans of care, training and development appropriate to needs were developed and delivered. The practitioner was also able to facilitate opportunities to work with staff from the community who had specific skills that the nursing home staff required. Community staff spent time in the home supporting staff in the short term to develop competencies and confidence.

The key overarching issues identified in the assessments were:

- Patients with chronic disease tended not to be reviewed on a regular basis by the primary care team as patients cannot normally attend GP clinics.
- There was lack of continuity regarding GP support as patients see whichever GP visits.
- Some confusion regarding diagnoses was evident with nursing home having a different understanding than primary care records.
- There was confusion regarding medication because in patients who had frequent admissions it was identified that the clinical records (GP) often had different medication than the home, and there were also some issues regarding compliance with medication regimes. Some patients were on medication that had been continued but on review was not required.
- Some lack of capacity and capability in nursing home staff which meant that early signs of deterioration was missed. This also included some lack of up-to-date knowledge regarding some of the long-term conditions in general terms.
- Lack of rehabilitation support when patients were discharged from emergency admissions.
- Lack of follow-up when patients were discharged, which led to appropriate actions required on discharge not always being delivered.

The community matron was able to provide both knowledge and expertise to manage the gaps in skill in staff that not only improved care and outcomes for patients but also *provided some development processes for the staff. The practitioner was also able to improve the communication between the practices, carrying out reviews of patients with long-term conditions. These included medication reviews that improved the medication compliance and reduced some of the issues that the nursing home had with patients who struggle with the number of medicines they are required to take. Emergency advice to the nursing home was provided in hours by the community matron and out of hours through the intermediate care team. This enabled an assessment of the patient problem, with investigation and management if required being carried out in the community, thereby preventing a hospital admission. The community matron was also able to arrange for fast track assessment of patients by the therapy teams, specialist teams and consultant in elderly medicine through the intermediate care services, which on a number of occasions prevented admission (domains A, C and F).*

The outcomes for the patients and the nursing home staff of the management as part of this caseload were:

- *Direct access to support when needed*
- *Reduction in emergency admissions*
- *Reduction in request for visits from primary care*
- *Reduction in out of hours calls*
- *Reduction in antibiotic prescribing in the home*
- *Improved medication compliance and understanding*
- *Improved communication with primary care*
- *Development of staff and improved skills, with higher levels of confidence*

Case study 2

Mr F is a 60-year-old man who lives with his daughter, his wife having died a year ago. Mr F was an active and independent man who had nursed his wife through a cancer diagnosis and palliative care. Mr F wanted nothing more than to play with his granddaughter and family, spending time with his friends, the occasional walk or time out with them was all he wanted. He was diagnosed with motor neurone disease and had a number of admissions following falls and a lack of ability to self-care. He had been informed of his diagnosis 3 months ago and offered support from a specialist nurse, which he refused. It was felt by the specialists that he had been suffering from this disease for some time but because of its gradual onset had adapted to the difficulties the disease gave. Mr F also has diabetes and hypertension. Mr F was referred to the community matron because he had been admitted as an emergency three times in a very short period of time.

On assessment the practitioner discovered that since Mr F had been given the diagnosis, he stopped his medication for diabetes and hypertension (domains A and C). This had led to a lack of control of both of the diseases. The practitioner on completion of the assessment of Mr F was able to identify his level of knowledge regarding his diagnosis and prognosis (domain H) and with this knowledge provide some initial support and specialist referral for support. This gentleman and his daughter who had struggled to discuss his diagnosis and prognosis, which had added further stress into what was an already difficult situation, should have accessed support. The practitioner was able to provide a broad range of information regarding the support that could be arranged and how the family could be supported. This enabled Mr F and his daughter to reflect on the type of support they would need at the end stage of his disease and how this could be delivered. This then allowed a plan to be developed to facilitate care being delivered to Mr F on the basis of his preferences and choice (domain H).

Mr F's condition had deteriorated very quickly following his diagnosis, but with some therapy support he and his daughter were able to develop some confidence in relation to his own abilities to self-care/manage and plans put in place to assist him with these (falls risk was identified and reduced, loss of mobility was assessed and managed to some degree, incontinence that Mr F was finding incredibly difficult to manage was assessed and managed) (domain C). Eventually after support for some 12 months Mr F who had been gradually deteriorating entered the end stage of his disease and was cared for in the end-of-life stage by his family, who were supported by the community matron and the community nursing service. These services were able to provide the family with the equipment and other support they needed in the last days of Mr F's life; he died peace-fully at home, as he wished.

Although the prognosis for Mr F did not change by the early interventions from the practitioner and other agencies, the outcomes for the patient and his carer were excel-lent. Mr F was able to maintain a certain level of independence and to make informed choices regarding his care right up to his death. He was able for some time to socialise and live a reasonably normal life doing things he enjoyed which he had stopped doing initially as he did not feel confident that he could do them. His daughter was able to give him the care he needed and keep him in the family home, which was one of his main wishes. The outcomes for this patient were very positive and while unfortunately he eventually died his family were able to celebrate that they could be there for him and that through the support he received from the community matron and the other services he was able to have a level of normality in his life for some 12 months, he was able to spend time with the people he loved and they were able to gather good memories that will stay with them forever.

Conclusion

Case management practitioners have the ability to utilise their competencies to make a real difference to patients. Outcomes such as reduction in emergency bed days and better resource usage are positive for NHS but for patients these are incidental positives. The real positive outcomes for patients are those that allow the patients and their carers to live as normal a life as is possible. For a patient just the ability to feel 'as good as they can' is a positive outcome. Patients whose disease has been poorly managed or symptoms badly controlled will feel an immediate sense of well-being if their disease is being managed and they are provided with good levels of support. Patients and their families can live with an incredible level of risk if they are confident that the support they need is available and will be there when they need to access it.

The domains reviewed in this chapter outline just some of the competencies needed in a practitioner who is able to deliver the support required by patients with chronic long-term conditions and their carers – informal or formal. It would be almost impossible to define the most important competence domain for case managers, as each of the competencies relates so closely to one another that all are equally important. It is impossible to describe how one competency alone would deliver all the outcomes required by a patient and their carers. But it is clear that the domain that contains the leadership competencies is key to all areas of practice. Practitioners and community matrons are expected to act as role models and provide mentorship and support to those who are training and developing their skills.

References

1. Department of Health (2006). *Caring for People with Long Term Condition: An Educational Framework for Community Matrons and Case Managers.* http://www. dh.gov.uk/prod_consum_dh/groups/dh_digitalassets/@dh/@en/documents/ digitalasset/dh_4118102.pdf (accessed on October 2009).
2. Department of Health (2006). *Records Management NHS Code of Conduct Part 1.* http://www.dh.gov.uk/prod_consum_dh/groups/dh_digitalassets/@dh/@en/ documents/digitalasset/dh_4133196.pdf (accessed on October 2009).
3. Department of Health (2009). *Records Management NHS Code of Conduct Part 2.* http://www.dh.gov.uk/prod_consum_dh/groups/dh_digitalassets/documents/ digitalasset/dh_093024.pdf (accessed on October 2009).
4. *Code of Confidentiality.* NHS. http://www.dh.gov.uk/prod_consum_dh/groups/ dh_digitalassets/@dh/@en/documents/digitalasset/dh_4069254.pdf (accessed on October 2009).
5. Department of Health (2009). *Reference Guide to Consent to Examination or Treatment.* http://www.dh.gov.uk/prod_consum_dh/groups/dh_digitalassets/documents/ digitalasset/dh_103653.pdf (accessed on October 2009).
6. Hatton C and Blackwood R (2004). *Lecture Notes on Clinical Skills,* 4th edn. Blackwell Publishing. Oxford ISBN 0 632 06511 7
7. UnitedHealth Europe (2005). *Assessment of Evercare Programme in England 2003–2004.* http://www.dh.gov.uk/prod_consum_dh/groups/dh_digitalassets/@dh/@en/ documents/digitalasset/dh_4114224.pdf
8. Deparment of Health (2007). *Mental Capacity Act and Guidance. http://www.dh.gov.uk/ prod_consum_dh/groups/dh_digitalassets/@dh/@en/documents/digitalasset/dh_078739.pdf* (accessed on October 2009).
9. Department of Health (2009). Listening responding and improving a guide to better customer care . http://www.dh.gov.uk/prod_consum_dh/groups/dh_digitalassets/ documents/digitalasset/dh_095439.pdf (accessed on October 2009).
10. *Department of Health & Social Care Inspectorate 'Care Management Guidance Social Care'. HMSO London.*
11. Department of Health (2009). *NHS Constitution.* http://www.dh.gov.uk/prod_ consum_dh/groups/dh_digitalassets/documents/digitalasset/dh_093442.pdf (accessed on October 2009).

12. Help the Aged & Picker Institute (2008). *Measuring Dignity in Care for Older People: A Research Report for Help the Aged*. http://policy.helptheaged.org.uk/NR/rdonlyres/ EFD769F8-930A-412E-B079-FD058EE6AA69/0/on_our_own_terms_021208.pdf

13. House of Lords House of Commons (2007). *The Human Rights of Older People in Healthcare Eighteenth Report of Session 2006–07 Joint Committee of Human Rights*. http:// www.publications.parliament.uk/pa/jt200607/jtselect/jtrights/156/15602.htm

14. Department of Health (2008). *Raising the Profile of Long Term Conditions Care: A Compendium of Information*. http://www.dh.gov.uk/prod_consum_dh/groups/ dh_digitalassets/documents/digitalasset/dh_082067.pdf (accessed on October 2009).

15. National Prescribing Centre (2007). *A Competency Framework for Sharing Decision Making with Patients. Achieving Concordance for Taking Medication*, 1st edn. National Prescribing Centre. http://www.npc.co.uk/prescribers/resources/competency_ framework_2007.pdf (accessed on October 2009).

16. Department of Health (2005). *Mental Capacity Act*. http://www.dh.gov.uk/prod_ consum_dh/groups/dh_digitalassets/documents/digitalasset/dh_080403.pdf (accessed on October 2009).

17. House of Lords House of Commons (2007). *The Human Rights of Older People in HealthCare Eighteenth Report of Session Joint Committee on human Rights*. http://www. publications.parliament.uk/pa/jt200607/jtselect/jtrights/156/15602.htm

18. HM Government (2007). *Putting People First: A Shared Vision and Commitment to Transformation of Adult Social Care*. http://www.dh.gov.uk/prod_consum_dh/ groups/dh_digitalassets/@dh/@en/documents/digitalasset/dh_081119.pdf (accessed on October 2009).

19. Department of Health (2009). *NHS Constitution*. http://www.dh.gov.uk/prod_ consum_dh/groups/dh_digitalassets/documents/digitalasset/dh_093442.pdf (accessed on October 2009).

20. Quality Commission (2008). *Standards for Better Health Care*. http://www.cqc.org.uk/_ db/_documents/Criteria_for_assessing_core_standards_08-09_for_PCTs_(amended). pdf and http://www.cqc.org.uk/_db/_documents/Criteria_for_assessing_core_ standards_08-09_for_acute_trusts_200903193552.pdf (accessed on October 2009).

21. Nursing and Midwifery Council (2008). *Standards of Conduct, Performance and Ethics for Nurses and Midwives*. http://www.nmc-uk.org/aDisplayDocument.aspx? documentID=5982 (accessed on October 2009).

22. Department of Health (2002). *National Health Service Leaderships Qualities Framework* (accessed on September 2008).

23. Carmel Hale Facilitator (June 2002). *RCN Clinical Leadership Programme: Progress Report for the North West Region*. (www.northwest.nhs.uk)

24. Department of Health (2008). *Inspiring Leaders: Leadership for Quality*. Guidance for NHS Talent and Leadership Plans. http://www.dh.gov.uk/prod_consum_dh/ groups/dh_digitalassets/documents/digitalasset/dh_093407.pdf (accessed on October 2009).

25. Department of Health (2008). *High Quality Care for All: NHS Next Stage Review*. Final Report. http://www.dh.gov.uk/prod_consum_dh/groups/dh_digitalassets/@dh/ @en/documents/digitalasset/dh_085828.pdf (accessed on October 2009).

26. Department of Health (2009). *High Quality Care for All: Operating Framework for the NHS 2009/2010*. http://www.dh.gov.uk/prod_consum_dh/groups/dh_digitalassets/ @dh/@en/documents/digitalasset/dh_091446.pdf (accessed on October 2009).

27. Wanless, D (2002). *Securing our Future Health – Taking a Long Term View*. Final Report. Department of Health. http://www.hm-treasury.gov.uk/consult_wanless_index.htm (accessed on October 2009).

28. Dixon A (ed) (2007). *Engaging Patients in Their Health: How the NHS Needs to Change.* The King's Fund. http://www.kingsfund.org.uk/applications/site_search/?term= Engaging+Patients+in+Their+Health%3A+How+the+NHS+Needs+to+Change &searchreferer_id=2&submit.x=17&submit.y=6 (accessed on October 2009).
29. Comprehensive Area Assessment Audit Commission (2009). http://www.audit-commission.gov.uk/SiteCollectionDocuments/MethodologyAndTools/Guidance/ caaframework10feb09REP.pdf (accessed on October 2009).
30. NICE (2004). *Improving Supportive and Palliative Care for Adults with Cancer.* NICE Guidance on Cancer Services. http://www.nice.org.uk/nicemedia/pdf/csgspmanual. pdf (accessed on October 2009).
31. NICE (2004). *Improving Supportive and Palliative Care for Adults with Cancer Research Evidence.* NICE Guidance on Cancer Services. http://www.nice.org.uk/nicemedia/ pdf/csgspresearchevidence.pdf (accessed on October 2009).

Chapter 6
Outcomes of Case Management for Social Care and Older People

Introduction

The implementation of case management across the National Health Service (NHS) has generated some discussion in social care for some years. Since the implementation of the care in the community programme during the early 1990s social care practitioners (social workers) have been undertaking a process known as care management. The practitioners were supplied with a range of guidance to deliver case management [1,2]. These guidelines define care management and the assessment that underpins it as being the cornerstone of quality care. The assessment in the care management process aims to identify and address the needs of individuals from available resources. The process highlights that the needs of a service user will be unique to the individual concerned. Care management is also described as a process of tailoring services to the needs of the individual. For those now developing case management programmes or competencies these descriptions will sound very familiar as they are reflected in the descriptions of case management. This chapter will review the policy drivers in relation to the care of older people since 2004 and then the potential outcomes for older people that case management competencies might deliver.

The number of older people in the population is continuously rising as life expectancy is rising and the standardised mortality rates are falling [3]; therefore, the number of people requiring care for long-term conditions and/or with complex support needs will grow and the pressures on services will increase.

Policy drivers for the care of older people

In March 2001, the Department of Health published the National Service Framework (NSF) for Older People that outlined eight standards, each of which had milestones for delivery [4]; a ninth standard was added after the publication. The nine standard areas are as follows:

1. rooting out age discrimination
2. person-centred care
3. intermediate care

4. general hospital care
5. stroke
6. falls
7. mental health in older people
8. the promotion of health and active life in older age
9. medicines management (added later)

Delivery against the NSF even with the milestones has not been fully achieved and the review of delivery against the NSF in 2004 reported poor levels of achievement in some milestone areas [5].

Following the publication of the NSF for Older People, the National Director of Older People's Health was appointed to lead the implementation of the NSF. He published his report in November 2004 [6], which described the progress in implementation of the NSF and the key drivers for service reform and the principles on which the vision for improving the health of older people had been developed. This report outlines a vision for older peoples' care that will sound very familiar to those working in case management. (Although the titles may be slightly different, their meaning matches the current policy exactly.) The vision outlined in the report includes:

- person-centred care
- joined up services (integrated)
- timely response to needs
- promotion of health and active life

The report presents some excellent practice via case studies and improvements in outcomes of care for older people, which includes reductions in standardised mortality rates across all disease areas, increase in health promotion activities in older people (increased smoking cessation rates in people over the age of 60, increased flu vaccination rates in those over 65 and increased number of women aged 65 accessing screening for breast cancer), improvement in service provision (intermediate care, community equipment, intensive home care, reduced delays in discharge both general and those over 75), improvement in services in acute care (90% coverage of specialist stroke services, increased coverage of integrated continence services), reductions in discrimination and improvement in attitudes to older people (established adult protection policies in 70% of localities, 80% implementation of single-assessment processes). The report also describes the further drivers for change in the care of older people, although it is clear that no further targets will be set in place to replace the targets in the NSF that were due to be achieved in April 2005. The report outlines a number of key processes for improvements in care:

- national and local targets
- developments in technology
- electronic personal care record
- independent health and social care inspection
- local older peoples' champions

In his second report in 2007, Professor Philip [7] outlined both numerical and financial impacts in relation to care provided by the NHS and social care for older people. In 2003/2004, £16.47 billion or 43% of the total NHS budget and 65% of acute hospital beds and in 2004/2005 63% of all finished consultant episodes and 58% (£6.38 billion) of social services budgets were spent on older people and 1.23 million people received social care packages. Successful services in a number of areas were reviewed in this report.

In 2004 the King's Fund produced a working paper [8] outlining a possible policy framework for integrated care for older people. The group that developed the framework the CARMEN network (Care and Management of Services for Older People in Europe) produced a set of national policy recommendations based on the experiences of members of the network from across the European Union. These recommendations were that national policy should promote development of integrated care by:

- Setting clear vision for services, which ensures quality of life, independence and control and improvements in service for older people with complex needs using a holistic approach to service design and delivery;
- Adequate resourcing, incentives for good practice, coherent regulation and inspection to promote integrated service models;
- Balancing service allocations, which are not directed at acute care to the expense of community services;
- Strengthening the integration between informal and formal care sectors, supporting carers explicitly in their role;
- Developing person-centred care programmes through which people are offered real choice;
- Ensuring the involvement of older people and their carers in modelling of services;
- Supporting the development of new care models through sharing good practice, supporting leadership development for staff and supporting the development of technology to assist people to remain in their own homes.

Many of these areas of policy guidance can be seen reflected in the current health and social care policy.

In July 2005, the King's Fund published the Wanless Social Care Review. [9]. The Wanless Review Team had begun its work by looking at the 2001 spending review by Derek Wanless, and clearly reflected that the shape of social care for older people in the future will be dependent on what the society wants and expects to achieve. The review utilised the Green Paper on adult social care [10], the public sector agreements [11] and the NSF for older people to inform its thoughts on the strategic objectives for older peoples' care in the future. It is clear in this report that the aspirations and expectations of older people are changing, with more emphasis being on choice, quality and preventing discrimination. The so-called baby boomer generation born between 1945 and 1954, who will be reaching their 70s in 2020s, are already exhibiting a very different attitude towards their later lives than previous generations. The review outlined the potential numbers in the aging population in 2025 and the possible problems this would bring. At the time of the report there was an expected raise of 183% in the number aged over 85 and 143% increase in those aged 65. The report noted an expected increase in the number of dementia suffers and fewer children to act as carers but more people with spousal care responsibilities. The report also highlighted a widened disparity between income and net wealth on retirement and inadequate pension saving by individuals ahead of retirement.

Health and social care integration

'Independence, Well-being and Choice' [10] clearly outlines the outcomes for social care in the future, which were derived from what the public told the government what they wanted. The outcomes are as follows:

- improved health
- improved quality of life
- making a positive contribution
- exercise of choice and control
- freedom from discrimination and harassment
- economic well-being
- personal dignity

The document outlines clear targets for health and social care to move on to a system where adults are able to take control of their lives, enabling them to make choices and decisions regarding their ongoing care.

The economic impact of chronic diseases is clearly understood [12]. Chronic diseases account for largest share of overall mortality across the developing world and there is a significant burden on the poor. In an attempt to manage this burden, the Department of Health has been focusing its policy on modernisation of health and social care. 'Our Health, Our Care, Our Say' [13] published following extensive consultation sets a clear modernisation agenda for health and social care, reinforcing the need for services to be joined up at the local level and further strengthening the guidance in relation to increased support for patient with long-term conditions. The vision in this document was outlined in response to the fact that the number of people over 65 year with a long-term condition is likely to double each decade and the 6 million people in England care for family or friend. The policy document reiterates the need to improve the health and well-being of people in England, and in fact defines the end point for this as 'to ensure that longer life means more years of health and well-being'. The policy document forms the framework on which the future for health and social care has developed since its publication.

The vision of providing services locally within communities in line with what the public request is further supported through the publication of the sister document 'Our Health, Our Care, Our Community' [14]. The vision for increased service delivery in the community is clearly in line with all policies for health and social care largely owing to the recognition that the NHS carries out a large amount of care within acute care that could easily be delivered within the community, the advances in medical technology mean that complex facilities for interventions are no longer required and of course it is the preference of the public that services are local and accessible.

The proposals in the policy document outline that it is essential that providers involve the community and public in designing and planning of services. Health and social care services should be integrated and partnerships developed particularly in relation to social care and education, and new services that are developed must relate to the rest of the health economy (the development of pathways). The configuration of services at the time of publication of 'Our Health, Our Care, Our Say' was seen as fragmented, and the overall aims of all policy guidances published in support of this area were to deliver against the following four key goals:

- Better prevention and earlier intervention: moving from a sickness service to a health service;
- More choice and a louder voice: ensuring people are in control of the services they receive;
- Tackling inequalities and improving access to a wider range of community services;
- Providing more support to people with long-term needs.

Fifty-four per cent of those who took part in the consultation exercise responded positively to the concept of provision of services closure to home even if it meant larger hospitals may merge, concentrate on specialist services or close. The guidance clearly defines the expectations for clinical and social functions that could be delivered safely and appropriately away from acute care. The view of the department is clearly that locally based services have a great strength in relation to their ability to be shaped and developed to meet with needs of local people and circumstances and that they can be flexible and innovative in the way they are delivered. The framework for reform of services including the development of community-based services, included arrangements for practice-based commissioning, choice, diversity in providers and payment by results.

Cost of care for older people

In England more than one million older people (65 years and over) use publicly funded social care and local authorities spend more than £8 billion on these services. Although some costs are recouped from users through means testing, in 2004/2005 this equated to £1.6 billion, some £3.7 billion was paid out in non-means tested benefits to assist towards the cost of care, alongside private spending of £3.5 billion on residential and home care by older people [15]. Despite this enormous spend there is little evidence that it enables the achievement of the government's aims (promoting choice, independence and prevention). In fact there is evidence that despite the aim to increase choice and independence, spending on care home placements has risen at a faster rate than home care. In fact in 2004/2005 almost 60% of local authority spending on older people's social care was spent on residential or nursing home placements against the reported wishes of older people.

The provision of care for older people across Europe was reviewed during 2004 [16]. This review provided an overview of funding and provision arrangements for long-term care for older people. Europe can expect the percentage of people over the age of 60 to rise from 20% in 1999 to 35% in 2050, and of people aged over 80 to rise from 15% in 1999 to 26% in 2050. The cost of health care across all European countries rose steadily between 1970 and 1980. The spending on health care reduced during the 1980s owing to tight controls on public spending. There is currently no clear correlation between spend on health care and the state of public health, which has led international experts to suggest that there is much room for improvement in both quality and efficiency.

There is in fact evidence that as the population ages, by 2050 there will be twice as many people aged over 85 but the spending on long-term care will need to increase fourfold, and if this funding is not forthcoming then older people will increasingly be called upon to pay for their care [17]. This report by the Rowntree Foundation identified that the current systems are inconsistent and despite good intentions of the system, which aims to ensure those who are worst off are supported, the older people with least assets or low incomes would have no choice over their care.

During January 2008 Caring Choices gathered more than 700 older people to access their views and those of their carers on how care should be funded in the future [18]. The question of who should pay for care has been subject to discussion and debate for more than 30 years, and despite numerous attempts to create a fairer system, the system still appeared to be failing older people. Despite the ever increasing amounts being spent on care, the demands on services have increased to such a degree that it has become more and more difficult to qualify for state-funded care, which is increasing the pressure on patients and their families to fund care. This review identified a number of problem areas:

- Present system of funding for long-term care is not fit for purpose: the systems were seen as inconsistent, confusing and unjust.
- The cost of long-term care will continue to rise.
- A portion of long-term care funding should be universal.
- Funding of long-term care should be shared between the state and individuals.
- Better support for unpaid carers is crucial.

The issue of support to unpaid carers is a key issue. The provision of unpaid care is important in enabling individuals to cope and for services to manage. In absence of the unpaid carers, who support many of our older people and those with long-term care needs, many of these patients would require professional care. The Institute of Public Policy Research has estimated that unpaid care in

England replaces formal services to the tune of £67 billion and this does not include the potential loss of earnings these carers suffer [19].

The debate in relation to funding for the delivery of services to those with long-term needs even today continues to tax the minds of policymakers in health and social care.

What do people expect in old age and how will these services be commissioned?

To deliver services that meet the needs and expectations of people when they need long-term care, they must be person centred, with sensible pathways designed to deliver the care to patients. During 2004 the King's Fund completed an enquiry into the expectations of care in old age [20]. This enquiry focused on groups of middle aged (50 years old) people to identify what they would require from caring services as they will grow older and the required care support. The report provided an overview of the expectations of care for this cohort of the population, which included:

- Access to good-quality services and information, advocacy and advice;
- Good-quality, safe and effective care;
- Facilitation of choice of care environment;
- Care within the community to support independence;
- Changing role of children and families: they will be less likely to provide care and support;
- Increased expectations in relation to individual choice and care based on their own needs.

There have been a number of reports that outline guidance on shaping services around the needs of individuals alongside a number of recent policy drivers in relation to person-centred care clearly outline the need for care for all people including older citizens to be designed and delivered in line with their preferences. Turning Point produced their report 'A personal approach to public services' [21], which is described as a 'call to action to those responsible for public services', providing a practical guide regarding what can be done to facilitate the development of user-orientated services that deliver good value for money. The need for commissioning of services by primary care trusts and local authorities, which ensures the delivery of targeted resources to those who need them, is a challenge for the public sector. The ability to commission services effectively in line with the needs of local people is assessed with primary care trusts via the world class commissioning competencies [22], and each commissioning organisation is required to improve its abilities in commissioning and the outcomes for patients/service users. Improved commissioning skills are seen as essential in the delivery of improved health and well-being in local populations. The review in 2006 of progress in delivery of the NSF for older people [23] and the supporting document 'Good practice in services for older people' provide examples of services that are known to contribute to improving the well-being and quality of life for older people [24]. The sharing of models of good practice in older people's services aims to ensure that commissioners and the service providers deliver efficiently and effectively the services that are needed.

The drive to ensure personalisation in care is supported through a number of policy documents – in 2006, 'Relentless optimism' [25] outlined the importance of commissioning in the delivery of effective and bespoke care. Patients and service users have highlighted their expectations and it is essential to effective commissioning that the views and aspirations of people who use services are part of the commissioning process. Commissioning is not about inputs and outputs but is about the outcomes expected from the service; it is about how service works across agencies and in partnership to deliver the needs of people with complex and multiple needs. There is, however, a challenge for commissioning personalised services as this is being implemented alongside payment by results, practice-based commissioning and direct payment arrangements. Whatever services are commissioned, they must be delivered in line with the expectations of service users, which have been described as being provided based on needs of the individual, being needs led not service led, enabling and ensuring choice, empowering service users, being delivered to meet the needs of individuals not targets and being provided by organisations who understand the people who use their services. The ability to commission services that facilitate and enable independent living, the right to participate in society and be in control of one's life is a fundamental expectation on those who commission both health and social care. As early as 2006, the King's Fund was offering guidance to both health and social care in relation to effective models of commissioning [26], which includes a set of key indicators of a successful market (ensuring choice, safeguarding continuity of good quality, encouraging innovation) and the problems in the current market such as commissioning approaches, nature of the industry, lack of consumer power, the labour market and obstacles to innovation.

What does case management offer to older people?

Case managers are skilled practitioners from across the spectrum of professions. Although nurses are seen as the key professionals in relation to community matron roles, all other professionals can also be provided the skills and competencies required in case management roles. It is essential that the workforce is appropriately skilled and experienced to deliver care to older people with long-term care needs. Case management competencies [27] outline a broad range of competencies all of which provide skills, knowledge and abilities to support the needs of people with long-term and complex care needs.

An adult social care workforce strategy [28] has been produced that identifies the competencies required in staff to ensure that services provided are appropriate to need and of course safe. The aims for this workforce strategy are in line with all the other policies and national guidances in that this has an expectation of a skilled workforce to provide care based on assessed need, provided by appropriately skilled and supervised staff that can facilitate and enable choice and independence, promoting well-being and dignity. The care and support service users will need will be heavily dependent on their health status and abilities.

Care delivery is a collaborative enterprise between individuals, carers, both professional and informal, and communities. It is essential that those involved in assessing service users' care needs should allow the service users to be a fundamental part of the assessment process; one of the processes that could be used is 'self-assessment'. The self-assessment process is widely recognised as a 'good idea' but how it is delivered is not clearly understood or defined [29]. There are a number of processes of self-assessment and at this time there is little evidence of effectiveness as the keys to implementation of self-assessment are self-reporting and self-completion, rather than examination and observation by a professional and some benefit for the service user. Self-assessment is being promoted as a way of involving service users actively in their care and empowering them to make decisions and choices in relation to care. However, it is important to understand that self-assessment does not necessarily lead to person-centred care.

Social care professionals have a long history of case (care) management based on procurement and co-ordination of care packages developed particularly for people with long-term and complex needs, and not only for older people. Within social care the case manager will utilise the single-assessment process to complete a holistic assessment that is appropriate to the needs of the service user. The assessment will provide an overview of the service users' needs, allowing the identification of risks and the development of personalised care plans. The care plan allows the procurement and co-ordination of care packages across a range of service providers, who may be statutory, voluntary or private providers. There is a need for the social care case manager to build good relationships across agencies and recognise when the needs of a service user require a specialist intervention. The key for social care is to ensure that the care plan is agreed with service users and carers and that all reviews and evaluations include a view from service users and carers on the effectiveness of the programme of care.

The delivery of care to older people across health and social care has many challenges [30]. There has been a lack of clarity in relation to expected outcomes; for example, service provisions including the use of personalised budgets are not considered with the family in mind. There has been little evidence of adequate integration of services, which impacts directly on their ability to deliver a personalised care model and there is a lack of involvement of communities in the development and shaping of services. The Institute of Public Policy [30] has offered some policy recommendations that are felt to offer opportunities to improve models of care and the outcomes they deliver.

Integrated models of care

The delivery of case management in social care works well in integrated teams; these teams are effective in delivering the broadest range of interventions, which aim to maintain independence and choice for service users. Fragmentation of services with loss of continuity places service users and their carers at an increased level of risk. Service users with complex and multiple conditions, and their carers, need services that are integrated to enable services to support them and meet their needs. This form of integration has been the main focus of all health and social care policies in recent years [31].

The delivery of integrated services is a guiding principle in health and social care policy, and the recent implementation of a pilot programme for integrated care [32] offers opportunities for services to develop the leadership they need to develop and test new models of care. Service integration is seen as a pre-requisite to delivery of a world class health system. This process is seen as having the potential to deliver improved outcomes for service users and carers. The pilot programme offers a process through which leaders in service can develop the skills and knowledge they need to deliver integration, which in turn will deliver improved outcomes and service user satisfaction; improve quality and partnerships; improve relationships, governance and risk management; offer opportunities for innovation; and reduce inequalities. The programme aims to develop a number of programmes led by clinicians, working across health and social care, including programme evaluation and sharing of learning and good practice.

Impact of case management on older people

A review of the actual impact of case management for long-term conditions on older people [33] reported on five outcome measures:

- hospital admission
- use of emergency departments
- length of stay
- cost effectiveness
- functional health status

This review of 19 studies of case management programme provided weak evidence in relation to impact on hospital admission and no consistent evidence of impact on emergency department use. Evidence of cost effectiveness was also limited. Functional status was improved in four of the studies with the remainder showing no adverse affects. Length of stay, on the other hand, was positively affected with significant reductions.

For older people with complex long-term needs, it is essential that case managers are highly effective and utilise the full range of case management competencies. The case manager in social care will utilise some competencies that are beyond the case management competency framework, but it is clear that there are some common competency domains that a social care professional will utilise.

The competencies as outlined in the education framework clearly define the area of delivery expected from the practitioners when they utilise the skills on practice. Care delivery closer to home as outlined in 'A recipe for care' [7] can be facilitated and delivered through the use of case management competencies. The key elements outlined are as follows:

- Early intervention and assessment of old age conditions;
- Long-term conditions management in the community integrated with social care and specialist services;
- Early supported discharge whenever possible and delivery of care closer to home;
- General acute care when needed combined with quick access to specialist assessment;
- Partnership built around the needs and wishes of older people and their families.

Each of these elements can be supported and delivered through case management. The outcomes delivered through case management can provide many of the improvements in care and support required, but case management cannot deliver these outcomes alone, there must be partnership with other care providers as without this the impacts will be reduced.

Case study G

Mr and Mrs G have been married for 45 years; they have lived in their family home for almost 35 years. Mr G is a retired businessman who had been in a very senior position. Mrs G had mostly been a housewife and appeared to be very dependent on her husband, who made all decisions.

Mrs G suffers from memory loss and needs ongoing support for medication administration to manage her diabetes and hypertension. Mr G is deaf and suffers from angina. The couple was referred to the social care practitioner as Mr G was struggling to cope with the care support required by Mrs G, and on review Mrs G appeared to be very anxious and frightened when Mr G approached her. The couple have two sons who live away from home and both had raised concerns about their father's attitude to their mother.

A full assessment was completed, which included an assessment of both the general and mental health status of both Mr and Mrs G; the assessment also included a review of the potential risk to Mrs G in relation to safeguarding. During the assessment it became clear that both of them were not taking their medication and that they were struggling to communicate owing to Mr G's loss of hearing. The case manager then spent a substantial amount of time agreeing a package/plan of care that the couple felt comfortable to accept and that was designed in line with their needs.

The risk assessment completed in line with the local safeguarding adults policy in relation to possible abuse, leading to a care plan that included regular support to the couple, which while allowing them to continue to be independent also reduced the pressure of ongoing care through provision of social care support and medication administration. The case manager arranged through a commissioning process appropriate support services, made referrals to appropriate statutory services including community nursing and mental health support and identified some social support that allowed Mr G to get some personal time. A regular review/evaluation of the package of care was carried out to ensure that the package was effective and delivered care to meet their needs.

The main competencies used by the social care practitioner are as follows:

- *Proactively managing complex long-term conditions;*
- *Managing cognitive impairment and mental well-being;*
- *Supporting self-care, self-management and enabling independence;*
- *Interagency and partnership working.*

The outcome delivered was improved control of their health, which included improved management of medication and their chronic conditions through health support. The anxiety and pressures on Mr G when managing his wife were reduced through support services, which also promoted a high level of independence. The care plan enabled the couple to manage in their own home safely and provided reassurance for the family.

Case study H: caseload review

This multidisciplinary team of a nurse case manager, a social worker and a physiotherapist with support team has a caseload of 170 patients across a group of practices. The patients are referred by either general practitioner or other professionals; the patient is assessed by an appropriate case manager depending on the rationale for referral to the service. All patents have an appropriate lead professional who is responsible for the development, implementation, monitoring and evaluation of the care plan.

All patients are assessed using the single-assessment process in line with the requirements of the NSF for older people, which allows all services to utilise that assessment process and set of records. Each case manager can access social care services utilising a social care budget or continuing health care through a shared budget arrangements. All the teams work together to set the parameters of care with service users and carers, defining outcomes and expectations with the aim of promoting independence. The team through excellent communication processes utilises the skills of all the team members' and as each has a specific set of specialist skills, the knowledge and expertise are shared as appropriate. Each case manager has therefore developed new skills and competencies; for example the nurse has developed skills in relation to rehabilitation and mobility assessment from her therapy colleague. Likewise the social workers have developed an understanding of falls assessment and of areas of high risk in medication administration, which has improved their understanding in relation to service users' needs.

The caseload contains a number of service users with mental health problems (mainly in relation to memory issues) and the team has accessed support through a local specialist service to improve their understanding and abilities to both assess and provide advice for support to the management of mental health issues. These new skills have enabled older people with mild-to-moderate depression to be identified, supported and managed appropriately at an early stage, thereby offering an opportunity to improve their outcomes. Each case manager leads on a specific area in which they have higher order skills or greater experience, but each is responsible for ensuring that all members of the team develop as appropriate in these areas. So the therapist ensures all the members of the team are capable and understand falls risk assessment and prevention. The social worker leads for safeguarding and ensures the team is aware of the processes and can access appropriate support. The nurse leads on medication and chronic illness and ensures that all in the team can manage medication safely and are aware of the potential for deterioration in medical conditions and how these can be managed. The nurse also provides advice and support in relation to end-of-life care.

The outcomes the team is delivering for the caseload, as identified through an ongoing evaluation, are as follows:

- *Improved functionality on most patients;*
- *Reduced number of service users referred into long-term care;*
- *Improved medication concordance;*
- *Reduced out of hours calls;*
- *Reduced emergency attendances and admissions;*
- *Increased planned admissions but with reduced length of stay;*
- *Improved service user understanding of their own condition;*
- *Improved service user satisfaction;*
- *Improved carer satisfaction.*

The case managers in this team are utilising all the competencies within the competency framework and utilising these to good effect.

Case study J

Mrs J is an 86-year-old lady who is a widow and lives alone but with good support from her son and his wife who live nearby. Mrs J has severe rheumatoid disease (osteoarthritis) and has had a number of joint replacements, both hips and one knee. Mrs J also has some mild heart failure. Mrs J has been well managed, but since her last joint replacement (knee) she has been suffering from severe pain and has had peripheral oedema of both feet, made worse by lack of concordance with medication. Mrs J's pain is not well controlled and this is causing some anxiety and loss of motivation. Mrs J has had five admissions in the recent 6 months following falls.

Mrs J is assessed by a social case manager following a referral by the general practitioner for social support and equipment assessment. The single assessment was completed and it was clear from the assessment that a specialist view was required in relation to pain control and medication concordance. Following a specialist view, a plan was formulated to manage her pain through appropriate analgesics; as part of this plan Mrs J's understanding of her medication was also reviewed and concordance with medication programme was encouraged. Mrs J identified during these assessments some areas of confusion in relation to the reasons for medication and how and when to administer medication.

Providing Mrs J with clear explanation and information in relation to her medication improved immediately the level of concordance while at the same time improved the effectiveness of the medication. A key problem for Mrs J was her level of anxiety and concern about her own care and a certain lack of interest.

The outcomes for Mrs J were no further admission, improvement in mobility owing to reduced oedema and increased control of pain and improved ability to self-care through improved understanding of condition. A mental health assessment was completed, which allowed some support to be provided to increase motivation and reduce levels of anxiety. Overall Mrs J and her family reported being much more 'in control of life' and better able to manage, they were also able to recognise very early any changes in her health and access appropriate support to manage the change, which generally improved the management of her condition.

Managing resources

The case manager is an important professional in the process for referral to services and the management of the resources across the care sectors. The case manager must have a broad understanding of the services in the area, and an understanding of the competence and capacity of a service ensures that all referrals made are appropriate to the needs of service users. It is also essential that case managers are sufficiently competent to ensure that they refer only those who require intervention and that resources are utilised in a way that ensures the effective management of resources. Although the case managers are unlikely to have direct managerial responsibility for most of the service provided to service users, they must be able to influence the quality of the services and promote appropriate care. The case managers should also be competent to support the development of services through an understanding of local needs, influencing commissioning or service planning or service/care pathway redesign.

Outcomes for older people

Older people have a right to expect personalised care that enables their dignity and is delivered to meet their needs. The policy context of care for older people is clearly one of independence and choice and how care services support service users to make decisions. Personalisation of care is all about ensuring that systems are in place to ensure that choice and control are available to each individual. All services are required to ensure that when needs are assessed the service user and the carer, if appropriate, are consulted and that the plan is agreed between all concerned. It is clear in all guidance that the individual's wishes and needs must be central to the process and the plan must deliver care for those issues that are important to the individual. It is essential that the discussions in relation to choice and risk are recorded carefully, which will protect the service user and care providers and will also enable clarity in relation to the expectations the service user has.

Effective outcomes for service users are highly dependent on the development of a realistic and appropriate plan of care that clearly outlines what the expected outcome is of each intervention. Setting effective care plans will require the service user to understand as much as possible the risks of any care plan and how the risks are being reduced or managed. A supportive decision tool has been developed by the Department of Health to assist practitioners and service users in the process of decision making [34]. This document also outlines the expectation that commissioners and providers should work together to create outcome-based commissioning, ensuring an implicit risk assessment and decision making, which empowers people to take control of their lives.

Conclusions

It is essential that older people with long-term and complex conditions receive high-quality and well-managed care. There is no doubt that the pressures in relation to both the care needs of older people and the potential cost to fund care are likely to be enormous. The ability of case managers to improve the outcomes for older people while still at an early stage of implementation is also evident. Case managers are an essential tool for both health and social care in the push to improve the experience of care for older people. Although service users have in many occasions outlined their expectations of services, the services have been slightly slow to react. New commissioning expectations and requirements as outlined in world class commissioning and the operational framework for the NHS in England [35], the NHS Constitution [36] and a wide variety of other policy documents are all clearly focused on the need to improve the outcomes of care for older people. The quality of care delivered to older people is fundamental to the type of society we are and want to be.

Each competency within the case management framework provides a set of clear markers for care delivery through assessment, planning, implementation and evaluation of the service user. Older people are entitled to expect the services provided to be based on their expressed needs and though it can still prove difficult for some older people to express their needs owing to either lack of confidence or lack of understanding, the support provided by a case manager could provide the service user with the confidence to take a greater part in the planning of their care. The outcomes delivered for older people may not always be the outcomes they expect in health, but the key for the service user is that the outcomes delivered make a real difference to their sense of well-being and health and of course their ability to be in charge of their own destiny.

The delivery of person-centred care is another area of essential practice in the delivery of high-quality care for older people. As the concept has become more popular with policymakers and providers, it has become more and more important that people who are dependent on care services are included at the centre of all decisions about how services are designed and delivered. The competent case manager has both the skills and the expertise to ensure that service planning and delivery is person centred through care planning and influence on commissioning and design of services.

Agreeing the expected outcomes for the care plans for older people is essential to delivering good care. Service users need to be supported in expressing their needs and expectations and in expressing their views during evaluation of service provision. In each of these areas, the case manager should have the ability to promote both service users' views and good outcomes for care of older people. Case managers can affect positively the care of older people using their competencies, and each area of competence provides its own specific area of skills and knowledge. The combination of all the competencies is the process through which the real impact on care is delivered.

References

1. Department of Health and Social Care Inspectorate Scottish Office Social Work Services Group (1991). *Care Management and Assessment Managers Guide*. http://www.scotland.gov.uk/Publications/2006/05/16081522/12 (accessed on October 2009).
2. Department of Health and Social Care Inspectorate Scottish Office Social Work Services Group (1991). *Care Management and Assessment Practitioners Guide*. http://www.twenga.co.uk/book/care-management-and-assessment-practitioners_3795550.html (accessed on October 2009).
3. Department of Health (2000). *The NHS Plan*. http://www.dh.gov.uk/prod_consum_dh/groups/dh_digitalassets/@dh/@en/documents/digitalasset/dh_4055783.pdf (accessed on October 2009).
4. Department of Health (2001). *National Service Framework for Older People*. http://www.dh.gov.uk/en/Publicationsandstatistics/Publications/PublicationsPolicyAnd Guidance/Browsable/DH_4096710 (accessed on October 2009).
5. Parliamentary Report 2005 *The Forgotten NSF: A Report by Sandra Gidley MP Liberal Democrat Spokesperson for Older People*, 2005. (www.parliment.uk)
6. Department of Health (2004). *Better Health in Old Age: Report to the Secretary of State for Health from Professor Ian Philip National Director for Older People's Health*. http://www.dh.gov.uk/prod_consum_dh/groups/dh_digitalassets/@dh/@en/documents/digitalasset/dh_4093215.pdf (accessed on October 2009).
7. Department of Health (2007) *Professor Ian Philip National Director of Older People*, 2007 *A Recipe for Care: Not a Single Ingredient. Clinical Case for Change: Report by*. http://www.dh.gov.uk/prod_consum_dh/groups/dh_digitalassets/@dh/@en/docu-ments/digitalasset/dh_065227.pdf (accessed on October 2009).
8. Banks P (2004). *Policy Framework for Integrated Care for Older People Developed by the CARMEN Network*. King's Fund. http://www.kingsfund.org.uk/applications/site_search/?term=Policy+Framework+for+Integrated+Care+for+Older+People+Developed+by+the+CARMEN+Network.&searchreferer_id=11485&submit.x=21&submit.y=19 (accessed on October 2009).
9. Wanless Review Team (2005). *Wanless Social Care Review: Social Care Needs and Outcomes*. King's Fund. http://www.kingsfund.org.uk/research/publications/securing_good.html (accessed on October 2009).
10. Department of Health (2005). Independence, Well-being and Choice: Our Visions for the Future of Social Care for Adults in England. http://www.dh.gov.uk/prod_consum_dh/groups/dh_digitalassets/@dh/@en/documents/digitalasset/dh_4106478.pdf (accessed on October 2009).

11. Department of Health (2006). *Public Sector Agreements.* http://www.hm-treasury.gov.
    uk/pbr_csr07_psaindex.htm (accessed on October 2009).
12. The Oxford Health Alliance (2006). *Chronic Disease: An Economic Perspective.* http://
    www.oxha.org/knowledge/publications/oxha-chronic-disease-an-economic-
    perspective.pdf (accessed on October 2009).
13. Department of Health (2006). *Our Health, Our Care, Our Say: A New Direction for
    Community Services.* http://www.dh.gov.uk/prod_consum_dh/groups/dh_digitalas-
    sets/@dh/@en/documents/digitalasset/dh_4127459.pdf (accessed on October 2009).
14. Department of Health (2006). *Our Health, Our Care Our Community: Investing in the
    Future of Community Hospitals and Services. Health and Social Care Working Together in
    Partnership.* http://www.dh.gov.uk/prod_consum_dh/groups/dh_digitalassets/@
    dh/@en/documents/digitalasset/dh_4136932.pdf (accessed on October 2009).
15. Derek Wanless (2006). *Securing Good Care for Older People. Taking a Long Term View.* King's
    Fund.   http://www.kingsfund.org.uk/applications/site_search/?term=Securing+
    Good+Care+for+Older+People.+Taking+a+Long+Term+View.+Derek+Wanless
    &oldterm=Securing+Good+Care+for+Older+People.+Taking+a+Llong+Term
    +View.+Derek+Wanless&old_term=Securing+Good+Care+for+Older+People.+
    Taking+a+Llong+Term+View.+Derek+Wanless&old_instance_id=180550&submit.
    x=21&submit.y=14 (accessed on October 2009).
16. Informal Health Council, European Union (2004). *Health Care in an Ageing Society:
    A Challenge for All European Countries.* http://www.minvws.nl/en/folders/iz/
    health-care-in-an-ageing-society-a-challenge-for-all-european-countries.asp (accessed
    on October 2009).
17. Collins S (2007). *How Can Funding of Long-Term Care Adapt for an Aging Population?
    Practical Examples and Costed Solutions.* Joseph Rowntree Foundation. http://www.jrf.
    org.uk/sites/files/jrf/2093.pdf (accessed on October 2009).
18. *The Future of Care Funding: Time for a Change. Caring Choices: Who will Pay for Long
    Term Care?,* January 2008. http://www.kingsfund.org.uk/research/publications/
    the_future_of_2.html (accessed on October 2009).
19. Mullen S (2007). *Care in a New Welfare Society: Unpaid Care, Welfare and Employment.*
    Institute for Public Policy Research. http://fadelibrary.wordpress.com/2007/12/23/
    care-in-a-new-welfare-society-unpaid-care-welfare-and-employment/ (accessed on
    October 2009).
20. Levenson R, Jeyasingham M and Joule N (2005). *Looking Forward to Care in Old Age.
    Expectations of the Next Generation.* King's Fund. http://www.kingsfund.org.uk/
    applications/site_search/?term=Looking+Forward+to+Care+in+Old+Age.+
    Expectations+of+the+Next+Generation.&oldterm=Developing+the+Care+Ma
    rket&old_term=Developing+the+Care+Market&old_instance_id=180545&submit.
    x=36&submit.y=10 (accessed on October 2009).
21. Turning Point and Dr Foster Intelligence (2008). *A Personal Approach to Public Services.
    Shaping Services around Individuals Needs.* http://www.drfosterintelligence.co.uk/
    newsPublications/localDocuments/PSRBrochure.pdf (accessed on October 2009).
22. Department of Health (2008). *Commissioning Assurance Handbook: Adding Life to Years
    and Years to Life.* http://www.dh.gov.uk/prod_consum_dh/groups/dh_digitalassets/
    @dh/@en/documents/digitalasset/dh_085141.pdf (accessed on October 2009).
23. Healthcare Commission, Audit Commission and Commission for Social Care
    Inspection (2006). *Living Well in Later Life: A Review of Progress against the National
    Service Framework for Older People.* http://www.cqc.org.uk/_db/_documents/
    Living_well_in_later_life_-_summary_report.pdf (accessed on October 2009).
24. Healthcare Commission, Audit Commission and Commission for Social Care Inspection
    (2006). *Good Practice in Services for Older People.* http://www.cqc.org.uk/_db/_
    documents/Good_practice_in_services_for_older_people.pdf (accessed on October 2009).

25. Commission for Social Care Inspection (2006). *Relentless Optimism: Creative Commissioning for Personalised Care. Report of a Seminar*. http://www.ofsted.gov.uk/Ofsted-home/Publications-and-research/Browse-all-by/Documents-by-type/Thematic-reports/Relentless-optimism-creative-commissioning-for-personalised-care (accessed on October 2009).

26. Banks P (2007). *Steps to Develop the Care Market: An Agenda to Secure Good Care for Older People and Carers*. King's Fund. http://www.icn.csip.org.uk/_library/Steps_to_develop_the_care_market.pdf (accessed on October 2009).

27. Department of Health (2006). *Caring for People with Long Term Conditions: An Education Framework for Community Matrons and Case Managers*. http://www.dh.gov.uk/prod_consum_dh/groups/dh_digitalassets/@dh/@en/documents/digitalasset/dh_4118102.pdf (accessed on October 2009).

28. Department of Health (2008). *Putting People First: Working to Make it Happen. Adult Social Care Workforce Strategy: Interim Statement*. http://www.dh.gov.uk/prod_consum_dh/groups/dh_digitalassets/@dh/@en/documents/digitalasset/dh_085661.pdf (accessed on October 2009).

29. Self-assessment of health and social care needs by older people. *Research Summary: NHS Service Delivery and Organisation Programme*, 2007. http://www.sdo.nihr.ac.uk/files/adhoc/30-research-summary.pdf (accessed on October 2009).

30. Moullin S (2008). *Just Care? A Fresh Approach to Adult Services*. Institute for Public Policy Research. http://www.ippr.org/publicationsandreports/publication.asp?id=605 (accessed on October 2009).

31. Glasby J (2004). Partnership working in health and social care. *Health and Social Care in the Community*, 14(5) 373–374 (Guest Editorial). http://www.amazon.co.uk/Partnership-Working-Health-Social-Better/dp/1847420168 (accessed on October 2009).

32. Department of Health (2008). *Integrated Care Pilot Programme: Prospectus for Potential Pilots*. http://www.dh.gov.uk/prod_consum_dh/groups/dh_digitalassets/@dh/@en/documents/digitalasset/dh_089370.pdf (accessed on October 2009).

33. Hutt R, Rosen R and McCauley J (2004). *Case Managing Long Term Conditions: What Impact does It have on the Treatment of Older People?* King's Fund. http://www.kingsfund.org.uk/applications/site_search/?term=Case+Managing+Long+Term+Conditions%3A+What+Impact+does+It+have+on+the+Treatment+of+Older+People&searchreferer_id=2&submit.x=15&submit.y=9 (accessed on October 2009).

34. Department of Health (2007). *Independence, Choice and Risk: A Guide to Best Practice in Supported Decision Making*. http://www.dh.gov.uk/prod_consum_dh/groups/dh_digitalassets/@dh/@en/documents/digitalasset/dh_074775.pdf (accessed on October 2009).

35. Department of Health (2008). *High Quality Care for All: The Operating Framework for the NHS in England 2009/10*. http://www.dh.gov.uk/prod_consum_dh/groups/dh_digitalassets/@dh/@en/documents/digitalasset/dh_091446.pdf (accessed on October 2009).

36. Department of Health (2009). *NHS Constitution*. http://www.dh.gov.uk/prod_consum_dh/groups/dh_digitalassets/documents/digitalasset/dh_093442.pdf (accessed on October 2009).

Chapter 7
Outcomes for Patients – Cancer Care and End-of-Life Care

Introduction

The provision of high quality care and support for patients with a cancer diagnosis and at the 'end of life' is key to ensuring that patients and their carers are able to manage at this highly stressful time. Owing to the improving processes used in managing the disease, cancer has become for many patients a long-term/chronic condition. The development and implementation of the cancer plan and its supporting guidance has delivered many improvements for the care of patients with cancer. When the plan was produced, England was reported as achieving poor outcomes in relation to the management of patient with most cancers, particularly when benchmarked against similar countries throughout the world.

It is clear that the demographics of death, the age profile, place and causes of death have changed enormously over the last century. In 1900 most deaths occurred at home and most common causes were infectious diseases and much higher number of deaths occurred in young adults and children. The majority of deaths now seem to follow a period of chronic disease, with 58% occurring in hospital, 18% at home, 17% occurring in care homes, 4% in hospices and 3% elsewhere. Dame Cicely Saunders the founder of the Modern Hospice Movement states 'How people die remains in the memory of those who live on' [1]. While for some years the delivery of end of life care has focused on those with a cancer diagnosis, the transformation of the management of many life limiting conditions into chronic conditions, it has been recognised that this situation must change. The cancer plan [2] and the improving outcomes guidance for palliative care [3,4] have been produced to improve the standards of care and types of services provided for patients at the end of life. For patients and their carers a good experience at the end of life is described as:

- Being treated as an individual, with dignity and respect
- Being without pain and other symptoms
- Being in familiar surroundings
- Being in the company of close family and/or friends

The World Health Organisation defines palliative care as 'an approach that improves the quality of life of patient and families facing problems associated with life-threatening illness, through the prevention and relief of suffering by means of early identification and impeccable assessment and treatment of pain and other problems, physical, psychosocial and spiritual' [5]. There exists much guidance and evidence that well-managed palliative care is both effective and well received by patients and carers [6].

Despite the guidance produced and the achievements of the guidance, many people continue to experience unnecessary pain and other symptoms. The end-of-life strategy provides distressing reports of people not being treated with dignity and respect and not being allowed choice about where they die. It is clear that the provision of end-of-life care to all patients who need it is a fundamental prerequisite in a civilised society. Many chronic disease clinical networks are reviewing how the end stages of chronic diseases are managed as the ability to identify when managing a chronic disease becomes a palliative process is extremely important.

The ability of services to manage those with palliative care needs is also fundamental to enabling the delivery of care out of hospital, a key policy driver for the NHS for some years. We also know that the NHS makes greater use of hospital beds than other countries [7]. This has been shown by research which reviewed the effectiveness of palliative care services in reducing admissions and out of hours general practice call outs [8].

Caring for patients through any treatment programme for a diagnosis of cancer or at the end of life requires highly skilled interventions. The development of cancer and palliative care specialists over the last 20 years has enabled the growth of an understanding of treatment programmes, symptom control and palliation. Management of patients through the cancer treatment is clearly shown to be more effective if clear processes of communication are in place from acute to primary care and if the programme of treatment delivered complies with best practice. Each area of cancer care has through the national cancer plan and the improving outcomes guidance been provided with clear guidance on the most effective programmes of care.

Palliation is clearly only effective if it can be delivered in a planned and proactive way. Reactive palliation leads to a lack of pain and symptom control and to a poor experience for patients and carers. It is fair to say that the competencies required within palliative care should therefore be easily found within case managers and community matrons because by definition these professionals deliver care in a supportive, planned and proactive way. In this chapter the competencies used in the management of end-of-life care through case management are reviewed and the outcomes for patients defined. The NHS cancer plan clearly states that 'the care of all dying patients must improve to the level of the best' and identified the need to ensure a joint care manager is in place so that the needs of the patient and carers are assessed and delivered through communication across the multidisciplinary team (MDT). This process of care management is seen as the key to delivery of high quality of care supported by appropriate specialist equipment and priority access to care including care out of hours.

Gold Standards Framework for Palliative Care

The production of the 'Gold Standards Framework' for community care [9] outlines very clearly the key proactive and evidence-based processes that enable high quality end-of-life care. The gold standard framework outlines the expected outcomes [10] for the patients and staff:

- The patient is comfortable and free of symptoms.
- They are safe and supported in order that a 'good death' will take place according to their wishes.
- Family and carers feel supported, involved and content with the care they received.
- Staff feel supported within the team and are able to grow with confidence.

The Gold Standard Framework outcomes are delivered through seven key tasks:

- Communication
- Co-ordination
- Control of symptoms
- Continuity including out of hours care
- Continued learning
- Carer support
- Care in the dying phase

The implementation of Gold Standards Framework across primary care teams tends to take place in stages over time. And though it is recognised much of the care is provided already by primary care teams, the formal implementation of GSF does draw together care into an integrated pathway of care and assists teams to identify potential improvements in care. The broad implementation of the GSF across the NHS is seen as an effective way of reducing the potential variations across the NHS in palliative care. The key to delivery of GSF is early identification of patients who are terminally ill and expected to die in 6–9 months [10]. The identification of these patients allows early robust understanding of the wishes and needs of patients and families. Early identification also enables early access to equipment and appropriate support through a system of 'flagging' patients for priority access to equipment and care.

While the GSF was originally developed to meet the needs of patients with a diagnosis of cancer, many organisations are now using the framework to support the end-of-life needs of all patients. This need has been highlighted in the recent National Health Service Framework for Long Term Conditions [11] which raised the profile of palliative care for patients with nonmalignant conditions.

Integrated Cancer Care Programme

UnitedHealth Europe during 2004 to 2006 completed a pilot programme of integrated cancer care within the NHS which reported in May 2007 [12]. The pilot programme was supported by the Department of Health following the publication of the progress report on the cancer plan [13] and the workshop that took place after the review was published. The workshop was used to develop recommendations for the creation of primary care nursing pilot projects to improve the delivery of care for patients with palliative care needs in the community. A key aim for the pilot project was to place an emphasis in the move of care from acute to community settings, which has become even more important with the publication of 'Our Health, Our Care, Our Say' [14] and the more recent review of the NHS by Lord Darzi [15].

The key areas for development identified in the progress report on the cancer plan were:

- Identification of gaps and systematic planning of care for each patient
- Improved communication and co-ordination between general practitioners and consultants
- Development of community-based services
- Improved hospital discharge planning
- Use of more effective information systems for tracking and managing patient services

The key vision for the pilot programmes was to improve patients' experience of care through better co-ordination along the pathway and reduction of unnecessary hospital admissions through proactive case management in the community, providing a delivery model for the improvement areas outlined in the progress report. This vision will also be incredibly familiar to any person who has been involved in or read anything regarding general case management as described by UnitedHealth Care as the vision is almost identical.

The pilot programmes commenced with an assessment of 'where are services now?' to gain an understanding of the levels and effectiveness of integration in services and an early view on the types of challenge the pilot areas would have to manage. It was clear from this early assessment that despite much good work there was little integration across services, with substantial duplication of effort and very unreliable exchange of data between primary and secondary care. The initial review provided evidence that the poor processes in relation to information transfer from acute to primary care included insufficient information regarding diagnosis and treatment, which affected detrimentally the ability of general practitioners and the MDTs to provide appropriate care and support during and after treatment. The prepilot assessment also identified the need for improved advanced skills within the community nursing workforce to allow the staff to fulfil a role of proactive case management in partnership with general practitioners. The issues identified clearly had a negative impact on care for patients and their families.

The development of the pilot programmes commenced with a review of the findings from the national survey of patients with cancer, which had been completed in 2004. A total of 7800 patients were surveyed with 4300 responding (55%). The findings of 2004 survey were:

- 32% did not find doctors' explanations of condition, treatment or tests easy to understand

- 40% of patients were not told about support or self-help groups
- 20% of patients with prostate cancer and 13% of patient with other cancers would have preferred more information about how treatments had gone
- 30% of patients with prostate cancer and 19% of patients with other cancers did not fully understand the explanation of how the treatment had gone
- 50% of patients with prostate cancer and 39% of patients with other cancers did not have a named nurse in charge
- 13% of patients with prostate cancer and 9% of patients with other cancers did not have their home situation taken into account when discharged from hospital

To ensure that the pilots were effective, clear objectives were agreed between the Department of Health and UnitedHealth Europe. The objectives were:

- To improve the quality of care given to patients with cancer through improved co-ordination of care along the pathway
- To assess and seek to reduce NHS expenditure related to unnecessary care and duplication of effort
- To improve the satisfaction of staff in all sectors with the care delivered to patients with cancer

In response to these objectives, UnitedHealth Europe developed a programme that:

- Built on existing work and resources within each health economy
- Apply individualised, whole person approach to care
- Use MDTs in primary care
- Use improved data and information to strengthen decision making and focus on the right of patients
- Focus on patients' desire for more information and understanding related to their diagnosis, cancer care pathway and cancer journey/experience
- Use standards and measures to create a systematic approach to care from diagnosis to treatment
- Collaborate with key stakeholders
- Ensure measurement of the results

Nine Primary Care Trusts took part in the pilot programmes. Although the programme did not manage patients at the end of life specifically, as the patients were transferred out of the process at the end-of-life stage, its processes enabled the development of skills in the pilot areas in relation to proactive end-of-life planning and management.

Preparing for the pilot programmes

The initial assessment of services not only identified many aspects of good care but also outlined a number of areas in which there were opportunities for improvement. The opportunities/findings are outlined in Table 7.1. The pilot

Table 7.1   Findings of Initial Assessments for Pilot Sites

Findings in relation to diagnosis

- Monitoring of referrals and follow-up by general practitioners was not consistent
- Not all patients with cancers were considered by the MDTs
- Not all tumour-specific acute trust MDTs had a co-ordinator available. The presence of a co-ordinator was seen as key to the effectiveness of the MDTs
- Communication of results of investigations, diagnosis and treatment plans from secondary and tertiary care to general practice was inconsistent
- Patients were given inconsistent information on treatment options, expectations for their journey and outcomes
- Patients lacked guidance and support through this stage

Findings in relation to treatment

- Acute trust cancer nurse specialists provide valuable information and support to patients but were not available to all patients
- The skills and availability of district nurses to support patients during treatments was variable
- Patients found it challenging to comprehend and navigate the process journey: waits for clinical appointments were long, clinics felt hectic and parking at hospitals was a problem
- Patients lacked guidance and support through this stage

Findings in relation to transition to primary care

- General practitioners wanted more information regarding treatment plans, course of treatment and response to treatment for their patients
- Health and social service were not well integrated.
- Lack of patient information integration and communication across services
- The skills and availability of district nurses to support patients transitioning from secondary to primary care was variable
- Patients lacked information on how to access services; they lacked clarity on who was responsible for them at this stage and so may have felt insecure about their transition from acute to primary care
- Out of hours service for some was unavailable or fragmented or patients may not know how to access them

Findings in relation to palliative care

- Some sites were not using the Gold Standards Framework and the Liverpool Care Pathway
- Patients couldn't access pain medication after hours
- Patients' wishes regarding end-of-life care were frequently not elicited: there was no accountability or process in place for introducing advanced care planning and care directives
- Too many patients were dying in hospital when their choice was to die at home
- Bereavement service and support were often not available

areas then completed programme planning and preparation, developing a core model to improve care. This core model had three main components:

- Defining the population – it was clear that the NHS did not have a national method for this
- Adoption of new roles for staff
- Process, tools and technology to underpin the programme

Delivering the pilots

Clearly defining the patient population was not easy for the organisations involved in the pilot programmes, despite a large number of data systems that included cancer registers and lists of suspected cancer referrals in some general practices, cancer waiting times databases in acute trusts, results of multidisciplinary meetings and the Cancer Registries and Hospital Episode statistics. Eventually the pilot projects utilised all of these methods to identify the patient cohort, which was then reviewed by general practitioners and cancer specialists (nurses and consultants). The next important process was to define the roles and functions required to deliver the model of care alongside a clear understanding of the competencies the practitioner would require to ensure they were effective in the role. Another key issue was to ensure the integration of the pilot programme with all other care programmes to reduce duplication and ensure that the transfer of care between programmes was safe and seamless.

Once patients had been identified, enrolment began with contact via the care trackers who outlined their role, which was to support the patient through the journey of care. This post holder acted as a single point of access for the patient and was able to communicate across all service areas, providing a central point of reference for co-ordination of the care programme. The pilots utilised a risk assessment tool to identify those patients who were likely to be the most complex as this allowed this group of patients to be referred to a community matron or Integrated Cancer Care Programme (ICCP) nurse who worked in partnership with the care trackers to manage the patient through their care journey. Those patients who were assessed as requiring less complex interventions were supported by the general community services and the care tracker staff.

All patients were subject to a full assessment of their care needs and a care plan was developed. Care trackers and ICCP nurses completed a regular review of the progress the patient made against the care plan, regularly assessing their needs and self-care abilities and providing education and support as required. If a patient was admitted to a hospital, the care tracker or ICCP nurse would follow up the admission and plan the discharge, and all unplanned admissions were reviewed by the primary care–led MDT.

Programme outcomes

The impact of the programme was evaluated by the Picker Institute; some 619 patients were included in the evaluation with 58% responding (347), 47% men and 53% women with an average age of 65 years, but the range of age was between 23 and 93 years. Eighty seven per cent (294) of respondents had a carer, family or friend, who helped with their care. The carers were spouse or partner (66%), 16% a relative, 4% a friend and 1% someone else. Sixty three per cent of carers (181 out of 294) responded to the evaluation. The responses overall were very positive:

- Right contact for care: 84% carers and 87% patients
- Access to out of hours: 58% patients and 49% carers
- 85–90% of patients and carers felt listened to, treated with respect and had confidence in the service and felt they got clear and understandable explanations to questions
- 65% of patients and 72% of carers felt more able to understand and cope with their health
- 80% of patients reported being definitely helped by the tracker nurses to understand information relating to their care and disease
- 79% of carers felt the service had supported and helped them
- 80% of carers rated the involvement of themselves or the patient in the planning of the care programme positively

The evaluations of the pilot programmes with staff and managers were also very positive, with most executive sponsors for programmes reporting that patient experience had improved. Staff responses included:

- Programme worked well and the outcomes appear to be good for patients, with the delivery of a structured care programme with much improved support and single point of access.
- Greatly improved communication within primary care and across sectors
- Staff were able to develop new skills and formalise ways of working

While the response rate from general practitioners was slightly lower (49%), they were also very positive in the main regarding the programme. The real benefits of the programme were improved communication between all involved in care, improved information regarding patients going through treatment, regular monitoring of patients and feedback on their progress. The GPs also reported that patients and carers appeared to benefit from the programme through improved support, knowing who to contact and how, improved monitoring of their condition and better continuity of care.

   The implementation of these pilot programmes was in the main very successful, but it is clear that small pilots provide only limited evidence of effectiveness of the programmes. United HealthCare do not see the programmes as prescriptive (implementation must be as they describe); their advice is that the NHS should take the evidence and learning from these programmes and develop locality-specific and appropriate implementation programmes. They clearly outline the need to develop the capabilities of the NHS in relation to collection and use of data, review the tracker role and implement, adapting the role to fit the requirements locally, and finally to recognise the potential of community nurses to positively affect the care of patients with cancer.

Case Management and ICCP

It is clear from the outline of ICCP that this is a programme of care which links directly to case management models of care. This should not be a surprise as the organisation that provided the programme of care is also responsible for one of the models of case management. This programme utilises most if not all of the concepts within case management, care co-ordination, assessment, planning, proactive management, communication across sectors and advocacy for patients and carers. This programme also outlines the need to risk stratify patients in programmes to ensure that the appropriate services are mobilised to deliver care and that those services are recognised as essential in the whole picture of care delivery.

Risk stratification in case management is a fundamental part of the process and is used in the ICCP programme as part of what is described as a Health Risk Appraisal/Assessment which when used alongside 'good clinical judgement' ensures that patients receive the 'right care, at the right time by the most appropriate practitioner and in the least acute care setting' [12]. Initially the pilots utilised a validated assessment tool that had been developed for frail elderly patients in the United States, but very quickly it became clear that the tool needed the addition of some cancer-specific information. The decision to make these additions to the health risk assessment tool was based on the number of differences in assessment scores made through the tool and the clinical judgement scores. It became apparent soon that the assessment tool was producing a high number of scores of 1 when the clinician was scoring the patient risk as 2 or even 3. Assessments made after the addition of cancer-specific information provided much more consistency across tool results and clinician assessment, which is essential to ensure patient safety and quality of care. The evaluation of the pilot programmes reports that the use of risk stratification–enabled equity of care across the patient population equity is defined within the report not as same service for all but as appropriate services for all. The risk stratification used within the pilot programmes was:

- Level 1 low-to-moderate risk
  o Site-specific cancer diagnosis
  o Stable condition
  o Low-to-moderate risk of unplanned hospitalisation
- Level 2 moderate-to-high risk
  o Cancer with or without stable chronic disease, stability during active treatment and/or remission
  o Moderate or high risk of unplanned hospitalisation

- High complexity, high risk
  - ○ Multiple symptoms associated with a cancer diagnosis and treatment and/or multiple medical/social/functional problems
  - ○ High risk of hospital admission, functional decline of death

Dependent on the level of stratification a care plan including regular review would be developed and this would be delivered by professional with appropriate skills.

Case management competencies – what can/should patients expect?

The policy drivers within the NHS in the recent years have clearly focussed on the need to improve care for the 15 million people living with long-term or chronic conditions, which would of course include many cancer patients. The development of case management models and the competencies for case managers and community matrons [16] has provided organisations providing care a process with which to evaluate the services they provide and review skills and capabilities in all staff and professionals within those services. Providers of care are required to deliver the Public Service Agreement Targets; the key target requires that outcomes for patients with long-term conditions are improved and that personalised care in primary and community services is provided, which will, the target expects, reduce emergency bed days by 5% by 2008 [17].

It is clear that in the main all the case management competencies are utilised in managing patients with cancer or at the end of life, but it is also clear that a competency in a number of the domains will have a greater impact on the care of this client group than others. The fundamental issue here is how the use of the competencies affects the outcomes for patients, be that in relation to how the patient or carer experiences care or the ability of patients and their carers to self-manage or maintain a level of control that would obviously include the ability to make informed and appropriate decisions on ongoing care and treatment.

The fundamental issue for patients is will they receive the care they need when they need it, and while all staff would claim that this is what they aim to do, the experience of patients is not always as good as we would wish. The NHS through its modernisation agenda clearly describes an expectation that the patient's experience of care, how the patient feels the care has been delivered, must be viewed as important as the efficacy and safety of the care. All current policy drivers are to ensure that this is central to both commissioning and provision of care.

The case management competencies that have been developed to support organisations and professionals to ensure they are 'fit for purpose' to deliver case management programmes of care provide an excellent tool through which professionals involved in case management can identify clearly the outcomes for their patients and through effective use of the competencies improve the experience of patient and of course carer. The competency framework describes in detail not just the skills and knowledge the professional will hold but also the possible impact this will have on patients and the delivery of service. No one domain within the competency framework is more important than any other, each provides a defined set of skills and knowledge that enable the practitioner to be effective.

Domain A is described in the framework as advanced clinical nursing practice and includes all the subsets of competence that relate to the ability of a practice to appropriately perform a comprehensive history and physical examination. This domain also includes functional assessment, diagnosis of a patient who is unwell, planning, implementation and review of therapeutic interventions, assessing the needs and preferences of the individual and supporting the individual to manage their medication. The final subset linked to this domain is the ability to verify a death which has been expected. The effective use of these areas of competency to support patients with complex care needs with a cancer diagnosis or who are approaching the end of life whatever the diagnosis should ensure that the patient is appropriately assessed and their needs identified and managed. The impact on patients and their carers should be well planned and care should be implemented with early recognition of changes in condition and appropriate management of those changes. The patient should understand the use of their medication, how it works and what problems or issue may develop because of the medication and what to do about these and who to contact for support and how to do this. Medication issues particularly for patients on multiple medications are well known to be a major reason for emergency admission to hospital, and these admissions can have a negative impact on patients and their carers and of course use enormous amount of NHS resources often unnecessarily.

Domain B is described as leading complex care co-ordination. This domain contains the subset planning, implementation, monitoring and review of individualised care plans for patients who have long-term conditions and their carers. Further subsets include co-ordination and review of the delivery of care plans, development of risk management plans to facilitate independence, development and use of communication systems to record and report, acting on behalf of individuals to present their needs and preferences, ensures the appropriate management of physical resources and the protection of individuals and preventing harm. This domain provides the competencies that would ensure the delivery of a wide range of services for the patient, ensuring that safety is maintained through assessment and mitigation of risk and protection of the individual.

The outcomes for patients with a cancer diagnosis from this domain would mainly relate to the provision of care managed across the pathway; that is, when the patient is transferred between care services, which for patients with a cancer diagnosis may happen frequently, from surgery, to chemotherapy and/or radiotherapy to ongoing review that may be joint or single, and then on for day-to-day care in primary care. Numerous handoffs are always problematic for patients because this is an area in which patients often report confusion and problems usually because of duplication of effort and lack of communication between services. The case manager as the leader for co-ordinator of care is excellently placed to improve these handovers and to ensure that primary care practitioners have in the patient records an up-to-date understanding of what the situation is with the patient, including progress on treatment and medication and the prognosis if appropriate. The practitioner should effectively assess any level of risk for the patient because the patient and carer will be safer and can be more confident of the care delivery if risks have been appropriately identified and actions taken to mitigate or manage these.

Domain C is described as proactively managing complex long-term conditions. The subsets in this domain are the ability to plan, implement, monitor and review individualised care plans, assess the healthcare needs and agree care plans with the patient, support individuals to make informed choices concerning the health and well-being, support individuals to live at home enabling independence, promote and enable partnerships between care teams, patients and carers, work with teams and agencies to review progress and performance and plan for improvement.

The patient outcomes in this domain would be the assurance that the patient and their carers are receiving a programme of care that is individualised to the needs of the patient – a care plan that they have approved as appropriate to their needs and that is being delivered effectively. The patient and their carer should ensure that the care plan is reviewed regularly with them and is amended if it is not delivering the care they need in the way they need it. For effective delivery, the patient should be involved in decision-making related to their care and should be able to make informed choices. The patient and carers should be able to maintain an appropriate level of independence and control over their lives and be supported to take some risks if they wish. The role of the case manager in this process is to ensure that any risk is managed and that the patient and carers are fully cognisant of the risks they are taking and have been able to think through ways in which their wishes can be delivered while ensuring their safety.

Domain D is described as managing cognitive impairment and mental well-being. The subsets in this domain, which are key to managing patients with a cancer diagnosis or approaching the end of life, identify mental health or related issues, provide referral to appropriate agencies and service for support as required, contribute to the support or care plan needs of the individual, enable patients to access psychological support and empower families individuals and carers to represent their views and organise and access appropriate support.

Patients with a cancer diagnosis and those entering the stage of chronic disease, which is palliative, are likely to need some form of psychological support. There is no doubt that this is a highly stressful time for patient and carers alike. It is clearly understood that patients who receive a cancer diagnosis need support from specialists, and most cancer MDTs will have a specialist nurse post that can provide some of this support. It is though unlikely that this will be enough in every case. It is therefore essential that any practitioner involved in the care of these patients has the appropriate skills to assess and recognise when a patient and their carers may need some psychological support and to provide appropriate support when they can and to make referrals to specialist support when this is required. The patient and their carers must feel that they can access support and advice when they need it and be able to voice their needs and concerns appropriately to ensure their needs are met. Psychological support is often a neglected area of care, and services may not be widely available, but this is an issue that can have an enormous impact on the patient and carers. Support to manage a poor prognosis is essential and every patient will have a different level of needs – some are well able to manage/cope with the information while others will be unable to cope and will require substantial support. A number of problems can happen in this area when patients and families are not able to communicate or discuss the prognosis and plans for care. These issues can arise from the patient not wanting family to know or from families not wanting patients to know. Whichever the issue the problems can be difficult to manage, and the case manager is well placed to support individuals to develop the strength and confidence to discuss these difficult issues because the end result of not doing this can be harrowing on all involved.

Domain E is described as supporting self-care and self-management and enabling independence. The subsets in this domain mainly relate to promotion of self-care and self-management and improving health behaviours. The key subset that relates to patients with a cancer diagnosis or entering the end-of-life stage is E1. This subset is defined as helping individuals to change behaviour to reduce risks of complications and improve the quality of their life. The case manager can support the patient with a cancer diagnosis through this competency to amend poor health behaviours that might affect their treatment and improve their health behaviours to reduce the impact of their disease or improve symptoms. The impact on the patient in this area can be enormous as it may enable the patient to manage their symptoms and improve their feeling of well-being even if it does not make an obvious impact on the long-term prognosis. Improved health behaviours for patients undergoing treatments for cancer (chemotherapy or radiotherapy) may well impact positively on the outcome of treatment for the patient.

Domain G is described as identifying high-risk patients, promoting health and preventing ill health. The key subset in this domain is working in partnership with others to reduce risks. The case manager will use this competency to identify any risks to individuals or communities and ensure these risks are reduced or managed. For individuals risk assessment in care planning and care delivery is essential because if the practitioner fails to identify a risk to the patient this will without doubt have a detrimental effect on both patient safety and patient experience. Patients can be exposed to risk in several ways and the practitioner must at all times be mindful of these risks while balancing the need to allow patients to make decisions that may expose them to risk, which is of course their right.

Domain H is described as managing care at the end of life. The subsets in this domain are focussed on supporting individuals experiencing significant life events and transitions and then supporting the individual to prepare for process of dying, supporting families and carers to prepare for the death of a loved one and supporting the family and carers to manage the process of bereavement. The patient who is going through significant life events will likely require a high level of understanding and support. The ability of professionals to 'give bad news' was for a many years seen as a major problem for the NHS. Since the publication of the 'Cancer plan' and the supporting 'Improving outcomes guidance' professionals within the NHS involved in cancer care have received specialist training in communication and how to deliver bad news. It is without doubt one of the most stressful functions a professional will need to deliver and the way it is done can have a huge impact on the patient. The level of communication skills a professional has makes all the difference. Bad news is never received without distress; therefore, it is essential that the professional is able to assess the impact of the news on the individual. The mental state of a patient must be understood as must the support process the individual has when he/she leaves the practitioner. The importance of access to support quickly and effectively for the patient cannot be underestimated because the worst possible outcome is that a patient leaves the professional either having heard half the story or having misunderstood the diagnosis and is then unable to access advice and support. In most cancer MDTs, the team will ensure that there is access to support via specialist nurses either immediately or very soon afterward and that the patient is informed how and where to access further support if required. In all cancer specialist areas giving bad news is always well managed the same cannot be said of other none cancer specialisms. The training provided to cancer teams has not been available across all areas, but the Department of Health are as part of the planned publication of advanced care guidance planning to improve access to this training. Giving bad news to patients and carers in the community environment is different because in most cases the patients and carers are well involved with the team. It is clear though that the process of giving bad news continues to require a high level of skill and it remains a difficult task.

Once a patient and carer have received bad news they will require support to define for themselves what the news means, and how they will manage the information and what further information they need. Good skills in a case manager should enable this process, and the practitioner should be able to effectively support the patient and family/carers to define what they know and what they need to know and how and from where they will access further information. This needs to be done as soon as possible as it is the unknown that is the most damaging and stressful issue for most patients and carers. The practitioner must also be very effective in their assessment of the psychological status of the patient because support may be required, and it is essential that this can be accessed if required.

Preparing for death and bereavement is not easy; patients will need to be supported in this and the competent community matron should be able to assist the patient and carers to prepare and if not to ensure that an appropriate referral is made to a specialist team for this support. One area that the community matron must be able to carry out effectively is the planning and co-ordination of services to ensure that the patient and carers receive the support they need to enable the individual to make an informed choice of their place of care. The ability to plan a programme of care, co-ordinating its delivery and ensuring it is being delivered effectively, is an arena in which the community matron or care management practitioner should be most effective and the outcome should be a high quality patient and carer experience at a time when well-organised care is absolutely essential. If the care provided to a patient during the end of life is not effective meaning that they die in discomfort or not in the place they had chosen because services could not be accessed to enable this, the experience will stay with the family forever and can make the process of bereavement very difficult as the disappointment with the experience can add to the pain of the bereavement.

The real need for competencies

The ability to deliver the care required to support patients with cancer through their care journey or through the end stages of disease, be that cancer or some other illness, is an essential requirement for care in the twenty-first century. If we cannot care for those patients at the end of their life when the care they need is usually defined a 'good nursing care' then we are in a strange place in the NHS. In recent years it has become very clear that patients feel that the NHS has become very good at the highly complex (intensive care, etc.) but has lost some of its skills in the delivery of what is often viewed as the basics. The competent case manager or community matron should buck this trend with the delivery of good care through co-ordination and standards setting.

Case study K

Mrs K is a 75-year-old woman who lives with her husband. She was diagnosed several years ago with breast cancer that was treated and for which she has been receiving regular follow-ups but because of her chest problems she had missed the last review. She also has some chronic obstructive pulmonary disease that was managed by her general practitioner for several years. Mrs K found that despite accessing the appropriate flu vaccine each year, she suffered frequent respiratory problems over the year. Mrs K despite good support from her primary care team and of course her husband has had four admissions because of exacerbations of her respiratory problems over a 5-month period partly because she and her husband are unable to cope during her acute attacks. Following her last admission she was referred to the community matron who completed a thorough assessment and developed a care plan. During the assessment Mrs K reported to the community matron some discomfort in her back that she had been managing with over-the-counter pain medication for about 6 months and that she had thought was because of 'old age'. The plan has been very effective in enabling management of her respiratory issues, but the back pain continues to be an issue so the practitioner arranged for Mrs K to be reviewed by the community consultant who following investigations informed Mrs

K and her husband that the breast cancer had spread into her spine. The community matron was able through discussion with the consultant to gain an understanding of the prognosis and options for management for Mrs K so that she could support her and her husband in deciding what treatment if any she would have. The practitioner was also able to access support for the couple via social care agency to enable Mrs K, whose mobility was decreasing, to cope at home without placing excessive strain on Mr K. Over a number of months Mrs K and her husband coped very well and were supported through some palliative treatment to reduce the increasing pain Mrs K was having. The practitioner was also able to support Mrs K and her husband to decide on where she wanted to receive her palliative care. This was done through clear discussions regarding services and options open to them with support to define what their expectations and needs were. The practitioner also ensured that Mrs K was included within the gold standards framework being delivered by the primary care team, taking an active role in the process through regular review and assessment of Mrs K's condition and regular communication between care services and the primary care team. Mrs K had clearly decided that staying in her home was her preferred option as long as support could be provided to her husband with her care and any symptoms she had could be well controlled. Mr and Mrs K were supported and services arranged (night sitters, symptom control, support with general care) – both social and health, which enabled Mrs K to die comfortably at home some 4 weeks after the plans were made.

Case study L

Mr L is a 78-year-old man living alone in sheltered accommodation. He suffers from heart failure and rheumatoid disease. The effects of his heart failure are gradually increasing and he is having more and more difficulty in taking care of himself. He had unfortunately had a number of admissions over the last six months, each leading to medications changes and different advice with no clear understanding of the expectation of treatment. Mr L was unsure of his condition. He did not appear to understand his disease or the long-term impacts; he was also clearly frustrated with the constant need to be admitted when his condition changed. Following a full assessment the community matron was able to provide Mr L with a clear description of his condition and what he could expect from the condition. The practitioner was also able to advice Mr L on things he could do to recognise changes in his condition and how to access early support to manage the deterioration before it becomes severe and requires admission. Mr L was also helped to understand that his condition was not curable and that the main aim of treatment was to maintain his comfort and reduce the impact of his symptoms. Through good support from his general practitioner, the community matron, social care and family, he was able to manage himself for a period of time, reducing the need for hospital admissions, and was also able to plan where he wanted to be cared for if and when he required palliative support. The community matron was able, when the need was identified, to arrange support from a specialist team to manage his breathlessness and fluid retention and then admission to a hospice that was nearby and willing to be flexible regarding visit hours for his friends and family so that he could be cared for at the end of his life.

Advanced care planning

The NHS has produced a guide for health and social care staff [18]. This outlines the importance of discussions with patients in relation to their preferences for care delivery. The guidance was developed as part of the 'End of life care programme'. It is expected that in July 2009 the government will produce 'Planning for your future care' that will outline the type of questions patient approaching the end of their life may wish to consider and to enable professionals to support patient to consider the issue of advanced care planning. The current communication skills education programme in place for cancer clinicians will be modified and delivered to a broader range of clinicians with intermediate and advanced courses to provide staff with the skills they may need. The ability to carry out these discussions and support patients to make decisions is a sensitive area and must be handled by skilled professionals and must also be carried out in line with all appropriate legal frameworks. The guide not only encourages the professional to incorporate the process into routine patient care but also defines some of the key issues and challenges for this to happen. It is clear within this guide that the legal frameworks including Mental Capacity Act 2005 affect the process, and as outlined in the competencies for case managers understanding of the legal frameworks in which care is delivered is essential.

Advanced care planning is seen as the process of discussion between an individual and their care provider irrespective of discipline, and friends and family may be included if the patient wishes. An advanced care planning discussion would usually take place in the context of an anticipated deterioration in the individual's condition that may affect the individual's capacity to make decisions or their ability to communicate their wishes. It is essential that these discussions and agreements are documented, regularly reviewed and communicated to key persons involved in the care. The guide describes two key processes:

- Statement of wishes and preferences – a range of written and/or recorded oral expressions by which the individual can, if they wish, write down or tell people their wishes in relation to future treatment and care. This may outline their feelings, beliefs, and values that govern the way they make decisions and this may cover medical and nonmedical matters, but the statements are not legally binding.
- Advanced decision – an advanced decision must relate to a refusal of medical treatment and can specify the circumstances. It will only come into effect when the individual has lost the capacity to give or refuse consent. It is essential that there is a careful assessment of the validity and applicability of an advanced decision before it is used in practice. Valid advanced decisions, which are refusals of treatment, are legally binding.

All adults with capacity have a right in law to refuse treatment even if a professional feels this is not in their interests, and a number of options are available to ensure that the individual is protected if they are unable to give or refuse consent because of lack of capacity. There is also clear advice in relation to referral to the Court of Protection, if there is a serious doubt in relation to the validity of an advanced decision. The Mental Capacity Act also outlines the requirements to support and protect patients who do not have the capacity to make decisions for themselves, including the need for independent advocates and procedures required to ensure the safe use of processes such as lasting power of attorney [19].

This guidance is useful to support practitioner as they work to deliver care to patients particularly those with degenerative neurological conditions, and it is clear that the ability of practitioners to support and facilitate advanced care planning required the development of some key skills and competencies, many of which are outlined within the competency framework for case managers and community matrons. Many of the case management models across the United States have similar processes and guidance to protect patients and staff [20–22].

Preferred place of care and delivering choice programmes

The end-of-life programme has been encouraging the development of any programme or process that improves the ability of patient to make an informed choice in relation to where they receive their end-of-life care. A number of programmes have been developed: the 'Preferred place of care process' [23] and the 'Delivering choice programme' [24]. These programmes define the process and support required to ensure patients and their carers can make informed decisions on where they receive the end-of-life care so that there is no need for an admission to an acute hospital at the end of life unless this is the choice of the patient and carers. The cancer plan [2] clearly outlined the need to improve service within communities to enable patients to be supported to die within their own homes, and the recent review of the NHS [25] also clearly defines the need for patient-centred service models of care, which are delivered to the patient at the end of life.

The ability of patients to make these choices is dependent on a clear understanding of the care they can access and the services being available as and when they are needed. The services must be flexible and accessible and must be delivered quickly with minimal delay. The services must be able to not only provide the care required but also support carers in what is a frightening and anxious time. The need to understand what to expect as patients enter the end stage of diseases be it cancer or a chronic condition is essential as the biggest fears for carers and patients is the unknown and what they can do to manage symptoms and issues as they arise.

Conclusion

Managing patients through a cancer journey whether this is a long-term/chronic journey or a shortened journey requires highly skilled professionals. The cancer plan and other guidance supported by the National Cancer Director Professor Mike Richards has set the NHS a clear expectation in relation to improvements in the care of patients with a diagnosis of cancer. The Department of Health has through cancer networks and other bodies produced a wide range of improving outcomes and other guidance all of which clearly define the need for excellent co-ordination and proactive support for the care of patients during their journey through treatment for cancer. The UnitedHealth Europe delivery and evaluation of integrated cancer care programme pilots clearly support the use of tracking and co-ordination as a process that will both improve the patients' experience of care and ensure that patients will receive 'the right care at the right time by the appropriate professional in the most appropriate place'.

The competencies used by community matrons and case managers are essentially the same as those defined in ICCP and are easily matched across the programmes. The main difference in the ICCP programmes is that tracker roles are defined to support patients who do not require the full support of a case manager. Not all organisations have implemented case management models or tracker models to support all patients with a cancer diagnosis, but some have included those who have chronic disease or who have multiple pathology within the case managed cohorts usually by default because they have been assessed as part of the high intensity users cohort. Some areas have implemented a case management process for patients with a cancer diagnosis and these programmes have delivered good outcomes for patients. Case management competencies are without doubt the basis for excellent care for long-term conditions and patients who have cancer. The ability of providers to implement the models of care for patients with cancer still appears slightly fragmented, which affects the effectiveness of care for this patient group.

The competencies of case management can be seen to improve all areas of care for patients with a cancer diagnosis who have complex care needs or whose disease has become chronic in particular as the disease progresses and the patient approaches the end of life. Although case managers and community matrons may not necessarily have all the skills required in relation to palliative care and are not necessarily the only staff required to support patients on a cancer journey, they do have the skills and abilities to ensure that patients are proactively and effectively managed and supported along the care pathway through assessment, planning and co-ordination of the care plan. Excellent communication across agencies and care providers both statutory and voluntary will ensure that patient and their carers receive the support they require to ensure that the journey, whatever the final outcome, is seamless and provided to meet the needs of the patient and their carers.

The policy direction for the NHS has for several years been a move towards care closer to the patients. In 2006 the Department of Health published a number of reports that were produced following a broad consultation with the public. 'Our Health, Our Care, Our Community' outlined for the NHS and social care the expectation to work on partnership to improve all areas of community service delivery and specifically outlined some improvements that could be made in relation to cancer services [25]. The Department of Health publishes every year its operating framework in which the department outlines clearly the expectations against which the NHS is required to deliver. In the main this document is aimed at commissioning bodies (primary care trusts) and sets out clearly the expectation in relation to the NHS. The operating framework for 2009/2010 [26] outlines the clear move towards the delivery of the Darzi review [27] through redesign of services to move them nearer to patients and communities and an absolute requirement to deliver a quality service that has the patient at the centre of delivery.

References

1. Department of Health (July 2008). *End of Life Care Strategy Promoting High Quality Care for All Adults at the End of Life.* http://www.dh.gov.uk/prod_consum_dh/groups/ dh_digitalassets/documents/digitalasset/dh_101684.pdf (accessed on October 2009).
2. Department of Health (2000). *The NHS Cancer Plan Improving Cancer Services in the Community.* http://www.dh.gov.uk/prod_consum_dh/groups/dh_digitalassets/ @dh/@en/documents/digitalasset/dh_4014513.pdf (accessed on October 2009).
3. NICE (2004). *Improving Supportive and Palliative Care for Adults with cancer.* NICE Guidance on Cancer Services. http://www.nice.org.uk/nicemedia/pdf/csgspmanual. pdf (accessed on October 2009).
4. NICE (2004). *Improving Supportive and Palliative Care for Adults with Cancer Research Evidence.* NICE Guidance on Cancer Services. http://www.nice.org.uk/nicemedia/ pdf/csgspresearchevidence.pdf (accessed on October 2009).
5. World Health Organisation (2002). *National Cancer Control Programmes: Policies and Management Guidelines.* Geneva: World Health Organisation. http://www.who.int/ cancer/publications/en/#guidelines (accessed on October 2009).
6. Borras JM (2001). Compliance, satisfaction and quality of life of patients with colorectal cancer receiving home chemotherapy or outpatient treatment: A randomised controlled trial. *British Medical Journal,* 322, 826.
7. Higginson IJ (1998). Where do cancer patients die? Ten year trends in the place of death of cancer patients in England. *Palliative Medicines,* 12: 353–363.
8. Grande GE (1999). *Does hospital at home for palliative care facilitate home death? A randomised control trial. British Medical Journal,* 319: 1472–1475.
9. NHS (2006). *The Gold Standards Framework: A Programme for Community Palliative Care.* NHS End of Life Care Programme. http://www.dh.gov.uk/en/Healthcare/ Longtermconditions/Bestpractice/Palliativecare/DH_4105215 (accessed on October 2009).
10. Thomas K (2003). *Caring for the Dying at Home: Companions on a Journey* (Gold Standards Framework Text Book). Oxford Radcliffe Medical Press. Oxford ISBN 1 85775 946 X
11. Department of Health (2005). *The National Service Framework for Long Term Conditions.* http://www.dh.gov.uk/prod_consum_dh/groups/dh_digitalassets/@dh/@en/ documents/digitalasset/dh_4105369.pdf (accessed on October 2009).
12. Department of Health & UnitedHealth Europe (2007). *Integrated Cancer Care Programme 2004–2006.* Final Report. http://www.dh.gov.uk/prod_consum_dh/groups/dh_ digitalassets/documents/digitalasset/dh_074955.pdf (accessed on October 2009).

13. Department of Health (2003). *The NHS Cancer Plan: Three Year Progress Report.* http://www.dh.gov.uk/prod_consum_dh/groups/dh_digitalassets/@dh/@en/documents/digitalasset/dh_4066440.pdf (accessed on October 2009).

14. Department of Health (2006). *Our Health, Our Care Our Say.* NHS White Paper. http://www.dh.gov.uk/prod_consum_dh/groups/dh_digitalassets/@dh/@en/documents/digitalasset/dh_4127459.pdf (accessed on October 2009).

15. Department of Health (2008). *High Quality Care for All: NHS Next Stage Review.* Final Report. http://www.dh.gov.uk/prod_consum_dh/groups/dh_digitalassets/@dh/@en/documents/digitalasset/dh_085828.pdf (accessed on October 2009).

16. Department of Health (2006). *Caring for People with Long Term Conditions: An Educational Framework for Community Matrons and Case Managers.* http://www.dh.gov.uk/prod_consum_dh/groups/dh_digitalassets/@dh/@en/documents/digitalasset/dh_4118102.pdf (accessed on October 2009).

17. Department of Health (2007). *Public Sector Agreements.* http://www.hm-treasury.gov.uk/pbr_csr07_psaindex.htm (accessed on October 2009).

18. Department of Health/The University of Nottingham (2007). *Advanced Care Planning: A Guide for Health and Social Care Staff.* End of Life Care Programme. http://www.endoflifecareforadults.nhs.uk/eolc/acp.htm

19. Department of Health (2005). *Mental Capacity Act Summary.* http://www.opsi.gov.uk/si/si2009/uksi_20092376_en_1

20. Kaiser Permanente Regional Health Education *Advanced Care Directive*, North California. https://members.kaiserpermanente.org/kpweb/detailPage.do?cfe=289&html=/htmlapp/feature/289healthdecisions/nat_advance_directives.html (accessed on October 2009).

21. National Hospice and Palliaitve Care Organisation (2006) *Advanced Care planning: Caring Connections.* New Jersey. http://www.caringinfo.org/ (accessed on October 2009).

22. Hammes B and Briggs L. *Respecting Choices: An Advanced Care Planning Programme and Quality Improvement Toolkit.* Wisconsin: Gunderson Lutheran Centre http://www.respectingchoices.org/documents/QIToolkit_000.pdf (accessed on October 2009).

23. Department of Health End of Life Programme *Preferred Place of Care.* http://www.cancerlancashire.org.uk/ppc.html (accessed on October 2009).

24. Addicott R and Dewar S (2008). *Improving Choice at the End of Life. A Descriptive Analysis of the Impact and Costs of Marie Curie Delivering Choice Programme in Lincolnshire.* King's Fund. http://www.clingov.nscsha.nhs.uk/Default.aspx?aid=4091 (accessed on October 2009).

25. Department of Health (2006). *Our Health, Our Care, Our Community: Investing in the Future of Community Hospitals and Services.* Health and social care working together in partnership. http://www.dh.gov.uk/prod_consum_dh/groups/dh_digitalassets/@dh/@en/documents/digitalasset/dh_4136932.pdf (accessed on October 2009).

26. Department of Health (2008). *High Quality Care for All: NHS Next Stage Review.* Final Report. http://www.dh.gov.uk/prod_consum_dh/groups/dh_digitalassets/@dh/@en/documents/digitalasset/dh_085828.pdf (accessed on October 2009).

27. Department of Health (2008). *High Quality Care for All: The Operating Framework for the NHS in England in 2009/2010.* http://www.dh.gov.uk/prod_consum_dh/groups/dh_digitalassets/@dh/@en/documents/digitalasset/dh_091446.pdf (accessed on October 2009).

Chapter 8
Leadership and Advancing Practice

Introduction

In the chapter, the aim is to review leadership its importance in the National Health Service (NHS) and of course its importance in case management as a model of care. There has been much written about styles of leadership and this chapter does not aim to review all of this information but what it does aim to do is look at leadership in general terms only using some information on models to develop leaders to support the discussion. Models of leadership are well established and range from the trait or great man theory, with leaders who are born not made, through transactional leadership to transformational leadership. The second part of this chapter will then look briefly at advanced practice, and the role of advanced practice in managing long-term conditions and achieving improved health outcomes for patients and carers. These twin concepts of leadership and advanced practice are fundamental to the development and delivery of services to manage long-term conditions including case management.

What is leadership?

The issue of leadership is an important one in all businesses and of course in the context of this chapter in caring services. All professional groups have an expectation of good-quality leadership to enable safe and effective service or care delivery. But what is leadership? What does it mean to professionals? What impact does leadership have on patients in relation to either outcomes or quality of services? And of course why is leadership seen as so important in relation to case management?

The NHS relies on clinical and organisational leadership, which is not just a managerial function, to enable the delivery of quality and effective services. Leadership requires the person (the leader) to hold a broad range of abilities, which include being able to enable, empower, influence, guide, conduct or set directions, and in professional practice it is an important supportive process. Leadership in the NHS is required at an individual, team and/or service/organisational level. To be a leader does not necessarily require the person to be in an official managerial role, though many managers do hold this function. Many excellent leaders are not managers, they are team members but they undertake leadership functions owing to their experience and credibility with colleagues or because they at a specific point in time are 'leading' a project or development or have the 'right skills' to meet a specific need.

Leadership must rely on followership [1], without it leaders would make no impact. Leaders are sometimes defined as heading for a horizon that the followers may not even see. The followers must, however, participate actively in the common vision for the process, and this concept of leaders and followers shows the inherent tensions in this process. Leadership according to Obholzer must be about having a vision, which is supported by passion and fervour, and the colder, hard-edged element strategy, the setting of goals. The 'strategy' thereby enables the delivery of the 'vision' clearly. These concepts can then be seen as essential for the organisational delivery of services and new models of care, such as case management. These concepts and abilities would also be required in leaders within teams and services to enable development and delivery, though the level at which these concepts present may be slightly different. Throughout organisational and leadership literature the idea of a 'good' or 'highly effective' leader appears regularly; what the leader looks like to the world is often described in personal quality terms: having a presence, being a people person, has the ability to make people feel involved and valued and/or has excellent communication skills. The discussions regarding how to develop leadership skills then often begin with 'are leaders developed or born', and while some of the personal qualities outlined in leadership models are personality traits, there is a view that these can be developed in future leaders through appropriate support programmes.

The core task of organisational leaders is to ensure that the core function of the organisation is always in the minds of individuals and also constantly reviewed in the light of external and internal changes. Therefore, leadership in organisations can be mostly focused on managing change. Change is an area that is constant within the NHS and social care organisations and, as this is so, excellence in leadership is imperative.

What does leadership provide?

Leadership appears to be extremely important in promoting and enabling the development and sharing of the vision for a team or organisation, and also it is essential that leaders are capable of explicitly defining those areas of delivery that are absolute and not open for debate for whatever reason. Good leaders can deliver the positive feedback to teams and provide the members with evidence that their participation is important, both valuable and useful. This kind of leader tends to be one who has the ability to mobilise others and make participation work in teams and across organisations particularly at difficult times when unpopular change is required.

Delivering good leadership in the complexity of a constantly changing environment like the NHS is essential and requires high-level skills of self-awareness, motivation, empathy and personal skills. Good leaders are able to understand their own and others moods, they are self-confident, can self-assess themselves and their impacts and have a sense of humour. Effective leaders have integrity, are open to change, can suspend judgement and think before action and are often comfortable with ambiguity. Good leaders are seen as energetic, motivated, strongly driven, optimistic and highly committed, with the ability to build and retain talent in their teams, promote quality and provide service focus. They also hold strong personal social skills, manage relationships and people well, are persuasive, can manage change well and are credible in teams. When teams are asked who is a good leader most, if not all, of these words would be used to describe a 'good leader'. The ability to engender in teams and organisation a sense of belonging and ownership through engagement and empowerment cannot be underestimated when identifying organisations or teams with high-quality leaders.

For many years, the NHS and the professionals have been attempting to identify the knowledge, skills and abilities required in a 'good leader'. Many professional bodies and organisations have offered programmes to develop leadership capability in both managers and clinicians. The King's Fund for a number of years has been delivering programmes, which have been successful in developing skills in organisations across the NHS, to develop senior managers, strategic nurse leaders and medical leaders. The modernisation agenda within the NHS appears to require leadership styles that are engagement and facilitation focused, that is the idea of leadership that encourages and listens rather than bullying and telling, and that allows delegation for decision making.

Leadership framework in the NHS

The role of leaders in the NHS can be very challenging and requires the leader to hold a broad range of personal and other qualities and skills to ensure the high levels of performance that are expected and for which they may be held to account. The importance of leadership skills has been recognised to such a degree that in 2002 the NHS introduced the NHS Leadership Qualities framework [2]. The framework was developed to deliver a range of supportive functions including personal development, succession planning, performance management and connecting leadership capability. The characteristics, attitudes and behaviours outlined in the framework are those that the leaders in the NHS should aspire to enable them to deliver the modernisation agenda within the NHS. The leadership qualities framework contains 15 qualities divided three sections: personal qualities, setting direction and delivering the service.

NHS leadership framework clearly outlines the importance of personal qualities and values and the role these play in enabling leaders to complete their roles. Self-belief, a positive can do sense of confidence, is seen as fundamental to being a leader rather than a follower. The features of self-belief are the described as follows:

- relishing a challenge;
- being prepared to stand up and be counted;

- working beyond the call of duty when required;
- speaking up if needed – this enables their integrity and motivation to maintain them.

Skills in leadership

Outstanding leaders display a high degree of self-awareness – they know and understand their strengths and limitations and are not afraid to use failure to learn. They understand their emotions and their personal impact on others, particularly when under pressure they know the triggers that they are susceptible to. The ability of leaders to pace themselves and to stay with an issue for the 'long haul' is clearly a key skill, supported by a tenacity of approach and an ability to cope with complexity. The ability of good leaders to enable a drive for improvement through a real commitment, making a difference to people though health and service improvement, is an absolute essential for services. The deep sense of vocation for public service, with an absolute focus on delivery and achievement of goals and investment of energy in partnerships, and an interest in leaving a legacy of improvement are all outlined in the framework as evidence of a drive for improvement.

Within the framework the importance of integrity, particularly personal integrity, in the area of self-belief is discussed. In the area of personal integrity, the importance of integrity is linked directly to the amount at stake within the delivery of services. It is clear from this description that the ability of good leaders to bring to their roles a sense of integrity in what they do is essential. Leaders will hold a set of key values they have built from their life and work experiences, which in the main will assist them in difficult situations. These values alongside a commitment to openness in communication, inclusion of appropriate people in processes, the ability to act as a role model and a sense of resilience in the face of difficulties, all enable these leaders to function effectively and protect them in the process.

These important personal qualities are supported by the qualities outlined in the setting the direction domain. This is the area that relates to development and setting of vision for the future based on knowledge of all contexts in which services will be delivered (political and social). This ability to set a direction based on political astuteness is underpinned by intellectual flexibility and the drive for results. Leaders who perform well are able to identify and seize opportunities for the future, making the most of all of the opportunities and being able to interpret the 'runes' regarding the likely direction of policy and need. They have the ability to use these insights to shape the culture and vision of the organisation or team and influence developments in services in line with needs locally. This quality is the key to change and development in services as it is here that the real transformational changes in services, not just the gradual changes we often implement, are outlined and described.

To enable a leader to function effectively they must be able to very quickly assess a situation or information, then draw pragmatic conclusions moving from a focus on significant detail to big picture to enable the shaping of the vision. The ability to use information from a wide range of sources is essential, as is an open approach to innovation and encouragement of creativity and managed risk taking. The most effective organisations are those that encourage creativity and allow managed risk taking; risk-averse organisations tend to find creativity difficult to manage. High-performing leaders clearly are skilled at networking, particularly seeking ideas and information locally and nationally. These leaders know what is going on through robust and effective system that gathers this information for them. They tend to use these networks to assist them in shaping their own visions and also in influencing others.

Political understanding and functioning

All health and care environments are influenced by the good political leaders who understand the culture both internally and across the wider environment. These leaders understand what can and what cannot be done when they set targets and are able to link the vision for the organisation or team to the wider agenda. For a primary care trust, this could be working with local politicians on key local issues for instance crime and disorder, health inequalities and the views of local people on service needs. It is clear that whether related to a team or an organisation, no area can stand alone – every team or organisation must understand the wider implications of its role on other teams or organisations. Health and social care, like most public services, are highly politicised; the ability of leaders in the NHS to function within the arena will become more important as we move towards far greater local accountability for the NHS.

Setting targets and delivering outcomes

The ability of a leader to deliver results and the drive they use to do so clearly relates to the motivation of the leader to improve services for patients. The delivery of outcomes and results is important to deliver against national and local targets including those used to assess organisations by external regulation agencies such as the Care Quality Commission. The leadership framework outlines the importance of personal qualities that are the core of the process providing within the leader the energy and sheer determination to deliver results. The ability of an effective leader to set ambitious targets, usually exceeding the minimum standards, expected to deliver an added value to patients is fundamental to a drive to achieve. Alongside this is the need to focus everyone's energy on doing what makes a real difference or adds value including taking all opportunities to use partnerships and new ways of delivering services to make a difference.

The final area of the framework focuses on delivering the service. It outlines the range of styles used to describe high performance including the challenging ways of working and emphasis on integration and partnerships. A key area is leading change through people; this relates to how effective leaders engage and gain support of others to ensure understanding of change. Good leaders share leadership and encourage others, particularly clinical staff, to identify new ways of delivering services for the benefit of patients. This process of engagement and empowerment is fundamental to the current engagement agenda in the NHS and one of the key requirements within the NHS Review [3]. Collaboration and facilitation of teams and partnerships is highly regarded as a leadership skill and enables staff and patients to work to identify barriers and blocks to service improvement and potential ways of managing these while also taking staff and patients on the journey of change as partners rather than as an audience.

The ability of leaders who are effective to delegate and be held to account and to hold to account is a key skill and organisations within which these processes are well established are both effective and innovative. Many of the external assessments of organisations in both health and social care require evidence of appropriate delegation and accountability as part of the assessment processes. This requires a leader to have the ability to set clear targets that are achievable and to ensure that processes are in place to enable targets to be achieved. The ability of a leader to hold to account effectively is dependent on a climate of support and accountability not a climate of blame. The leaders must also be prepared to be held accountable for what they have agreed to do as a leader.

Empowerment and influencing

Empowerment of others through ongoing development is essential for the development of services and a good leader will support these processes. The features of a leader in this area are:

- An ability to work in the background, creating space for others to lead;
- An ability to spot potential and support development;
- Personal responsibility for diversity;
- Fostering development of others in the community;
- Engagement of service users and developing equal, open and power-sharing relationships with users to enable service developments that truly reflect the wishes of patients.

The ability of leaders in the NHS to effectively influence is highly important. The ability to influence strategically is a skill that was seldom seen in leadership roles inside the NHS; however, this is changing. Effective leaders are those who make things happen though the use of their influence. The ability to influence strategically requires a leader to obtain results through partnership working both internally and externally. This also requires an ability to cope with high levels of ambiguity as organisations change, and to identify the critical relationships and to influence these relationships using a range of influencing strategies to ensure effectiveness. This combination of effective and strategic influencing with empowering of others is seen as ensuring the health agenda is delivered and owned locally in the organisation, by staff and by local people.

The ability of good leaders to work with a range of internal and external stakeholder in partnership or collaboration is an essential requirement in a modern NHS. The requirement within World Class Commissioning [4] to develop within primary care organisations Strategic Commissioning Plans, which have been subject to consultation with all local stakeholders (both providers and users), is evidence of the push from the centre for increased local engagement and accountability. The need to understand and respond to diverse viewpoints and manage expectations is clearly important and can also be a very difficult circle to square. It is a key requirement that leaders in the NHS, whatever their levels of influence, are able to create successful partnerships across services and with users. At a local team level the ability of leaders in teams to develop processes of engagement with their staff and users of their service is equally important to the involvement in strategic plans.

Levels of competence

For each of the areas, there is within the framework a description of levels of competence, which describe the way the quality will present from level 0 up to level 4. The framework enables a clear definition of the expected actions seen in leaders and also allows assessment of the skills and capabilities the leader holds to enable ongoing development and improvement of skills. The framework is designed to cover all leadership roles and many of the levels of achievement related to the skills expected within very senior role, for example a chief executive, but the outlines can be useful for all other leadership roles. It is also clear that in certain situations the qualities required in a leader may be different in either level or approach. The situation leaders find themselves in clearly influences what they do and how they do it, but in all situations a drive for results, influencing and leading change through people are seen as highly important qualities.

Other leadership frameworks

The Modernising Leadership Model developed by NHS North West [5] provides a further tool that describes the behaviours that are consistently demonstrated by the most effective leaders (and managers). Although this tool is aimed at middle, senior and executive/board levels, its does offer developmental advice and support to all who seek to lead modernisation or changing practice within a service of the NHS. The model is not designed to offer professional or clinical knowledge and expertise but focuses on effective leadership behaviours. This model incorporates the leadership framework outlined earlier, further developing some of the aspects based on discussions with consistently high-performing leaders throughout the NHS in the North West. This model describes three levels of performance in behaviours and offers a clear description of what these levels will look like together with some tools for competency-based interviews and feedback via 360°. The tool therefore aims to assist in assessing potential and support development and training, provide criteria for systematic recruitment and selection and provide a framework for performance management.

The tool outlines the four key arenas that are essential for effective leadership:

- motivation
- decision making
- personal resources (personal attributes)
- working across boundaries

There are then three areas described as breadth of control:

- task delivery (team focused)
- process of implementation (multiteam)
- policy and strategy (organisational and cross-organisational)

There are then three levels:

- Level 1: blue
- Level 2: red
- Level 3: purple

The model therefore works in 4 arenas and 12 competencies – 3 in each arena – and behavioural indicators, each providing a clear definition of the behaviours that make the real difference.

In the arena of motivation the competencies are releasing talent, team enabling and articulating the visions. For each competency there are behavioural indicators. Releasing the talent requires developing performance, raising performance and empowering. Team enabling requires supporting teamwork, energising teamwork and inspiring teamwork. Articulating the vision requires aligning goals, building belief and envisioning the future. It is easy therefore to envision how at any level of an organisation these leadership behaviours could support the staff, service or organisation to make a real difference.

In the arena of decision making the competencies are analytical insight, innovation and creativity and understanding the context. As before each competency has defined behavioural indicators. Analytical insight requires analysing information, making connections and understanding complexity. Innovation and creativity require thinking differently, pursuing creativity and releasing creativity. For understanding the context, the behaviours required are board perspective, strategic awareness and environmental sensitivity. Each of these behaviours and competencies also has clear relevance at all levels of organisations and partnerships and a leader who can exhibit these is an effective leader.

The concept of personal resources is the arena within the framework in which the personal resilience and values are reflected. The competencies in this arena are responsiveness and flexibility, embodying values and achieving delivery. The behaviours beneath the competency responsiveness and flexibility are responding to the change, exploiting opportunities and acting as change agent. For embodying values the behaviours are living the values, modelling the values and serving the public. For achieving delivery the behaviours are focusing on effort, pursuing results and enabling pace.

For the arena working across boundaries the competencies are sharing information, building valued relationships and influencing change. Sharing information behaviours relate to abilities to communicate internally, externally and community wide. For building valued relationships the behaviours are networking, working in partnerships and creating synergies. For influencing change the behaviours required are clarification of views and the ability to win people over and change perspectives.

This framework clearly reflects the behaviours and competencies outlined in the NHS Leadership Framework. What it also does is provide information for those who wish to or are required to act in leadership roles on the sorts of behaviours they must either develop or consolidate to be effective and the levels at which the behaviours will be required if they wish their leadership role to have a wider impact.

Many other frameworks are available across the NHS and social care, these include:

- Leading in Empowered Organisations (LEO) [6];
- Royal College of Nursing (RCN) leadership programme [7];
- King's Fund programmes: Strategic Nursing Leaders [8], Senior Manager Programmes and Medical Director Programme;
- Leadership at the point of care Modernisation Agency;
- Inhouse (organisational) leadership programmes including action learning sets.

Most of these are specific to roles, for example the RCN and LEO programmes are focused on clinical staff and understanding how they can fulfil their professional and team leadership function and influence wider agendas. The King's Fund programmes tend to focus on developing strategic leadership functions in senior managers and director roles. For example, the King's Fund Strategic Nursing Leaders programme attempts to enhance the leadership capability by building on characteristics such as being a strategist, being politically astute operator, being a confident leader and having a sense of purpose. All of these characteristics link directly to those outlined in other frameworks, though functioning at the higher level of expectation as should be expected of nursing leaders working strategically in organisations or locally and nationally.

What does good leadership do?

Leadership to support learning and development in organisations and/or teams is a key function for case managers particularly. This requires leaders and managers to act as champions and role models for teams, provide opportunities for learning and development and build and support learning processes. The ability of organisations and services/teams to become effective learners is supported through facilitative leadership; this type of leader 'leads from the shoulder' rather than from the front [9]. Facilitative leadership makes people feel valued – it enables participation, helps to develop people and provides incentives. Learning for organisations is essential and is expected in organisations, particularly those in the NHS.

Leaders can be seen as those who, irrespective of their level or professional background, can influence people [10]. Transformational leadership defined as the ability to enable everyone to be a leader on something, through inspiring staff to believe in a vision for the future, challenging and stimulating, developing trust and communicating. This transformational model of leadership has replaced the model of transactional leadership, defined as making rational decisions and managing options. The focus of the NHS is now on transformational leadership owing to the need for leaders to manage in an agenda and organisations which are constantly changing [11]. The transformational leadership type requires what is defined as emotional intelligence [12]. This type of leader is seen as having a positive impact on staff, services and the organisation through an ability to inspire and motivate the organisation to deliver a vision for the future.

Impact on organisations

The impact on organisations, services, teams and individuals of good leadership is wide – a good leader will positively affect performance, identity and ethos [13]. The RCN review described that effective nurse leadership at board level would interpret and translate nursing issues and values into corporate objectives, influence decision making in a facilitative way and support bottom up approaches for developing strategy very much in line with the current expectations of the modern NHS. The skills in these nurse leaders were seen as consistent with transformational leadership styles, that is being democratic, developmental, engaging and devolving.

It is clear the good leadership develops people, so in services good leadership will develop the team/staff but will also support the development of users through empowerment and provide support for choice and self-care. It is also clear that transformational leadership styles that are more participatory are essential to enabling the transformation of services and care that is expected in the Darzi Review [3].

Effective leadership will always underpin development and innovation, for the NHS leadership must always be about meeting the needs of local populations, developing patient-centred services, interaction and partnership with other agencies involved in care/service delivery and the ability to be flexible in how services are planned and delivered. No matter how complex an organisation or system is, effective leaders will enable it to function through collaboration, cooperation and communication.

It is also clear from policy and guidance that high performance from leaders is essential in delivering patient safety; this is evident when reviewing success in organisations in relation to health care acquired infections, learning from incidents and complaints and development of fair blame cultures within organisations. The ability of an organisation to be patient focused and ensure patient safety relies on the leadership of the organisation promoting a culture in which incidents are reported and learning identified, where staff feel safe to raise issues (whistle blowing) and where patients feel they can raise complaints or comments and have these managed appropriately without fear of any negative impact. Weak leadership will have a negative impact on the ability of clinicians to argue for safe practice and raise concerns. The ability of clinical leaders to make an independent judgement on the safety of care is fundamentally important but the confidence of these clinical leaders to do something with information regarding potential problems with patient safety is heavily dependent on the strength of leadership in the organisation [13].

'Modernising nursing careers' [14] outlines in one of its priority areas the need to 'prepare nurses to lead in a changed healthcare system'. The leadership role that nurses will play in developing quality services that are patient centred and facilitate choice is clearly outlined in this document. It also outlines the need for nurses to develop leadership skills in relation to skill-mixed teams, maximising the contribution of all team members to patient care of particular relevance when looking at long-term condition services. Local clinical leadership affects the highest number of staff and should bring local knowledge to decision making, generate new ideas (innovation), develop and maintain standards and translate policy and strategy into reality [15].

Leadership in case management

Case management requires effective leadership for both its development and its delivery. The Modernisation Agency [16] in its self-assessment tool for long-term conditions highlights the importance of leadership when assessing the state of readiness of an organisation that is developing services to manage long-term conditions. The standards they expect of leadership relate to the presence of clear leadership for improving long-term conditions management, the presence of a clear strategy or vision of the way forward and all alternative models of care being considered. Evidence that the organisation at a senior level has reviewed all evidence for service models including the impact for staffing is required as this is important in ensuring effective implementation. Communication of the vision and strategy with broad range of stakeholders (a key characteristic of good leadership) is also seen as essential to effective implementation. The review of the experience of programme and clinical leads for the implementation of the Evercare programme [17] highlighted the need for the leaders, both managerial and clinical, to develop with all involved staff and service users and share widely the vision for the management of chronic conditions as for the programmes to be effective all stakeholders need to be effectively engaged and committed to the process. The ability of leaders to develop enthusiasm in staff and service users is highly important as this promotes concordance with programmes by both users and staff.

Leadership in the complex systems that care for patients with long-term conditions is located in the relationships and a shared wish to deliver on a shared endeavour for the benefit of users and carers. It is clearly the role of leaders to tell a good story to explain their vision as if the story engages staff it is more likely they will understand and work towards the vision. The need to engage staff, users and communities in the vision for a service cannot be underestimated as their understanding and commitment are the bedrock of success for the vision. The development of case management processes requires transformational leadership as this is about managing change in service models across organisational boundaries and integrating systems. The need to create partnerships to underpin both the development and delivery of process to manage long-term conditions is fundamental to success, and therefore leading for improvement depends on ambition and partnership.

Leadership and change

To be successful, there is a need for leaders to have the ability to change and act as a role model for others alongside an understanding of the context and culture of the systems they are working with. These concepts together with the ability to build partnerships, and build capacity through development and learning, make connections between values and beliefs and change, negotiate, influence, develop networks and focus on delivery of improvements for users are absolutely essential to enable effective change to be achieved. Case managers will in practice also need high levels of leadership skills; they need these skills to influence service standards, to influence and negotiate with providers of care for care packages and to lead teams that are multiprofessional and cross-organisational [18]. The leadership required from case managers is both decisive in term of making things happen and also receptive and reflective to the wishes of users and colleagues in the system. This system of care requires the leader (case manager) to influence without absolute control and to work in effective partnerships with colleagues and users. The ability of a case manager to work across boundaries and orchestrate care for the patients is a key requirement for effective care and improved outcomes.

The leadership role of a case manager is defined in the educational framework and in all job descriptions. The leadership functions required are developmental in relation to the model of service: leading processes to develop the services and develop and implement changes in clinical practice including challenge professional and organisational boundaries to promote improved service effectiveness. The case manager must also deliver leadership functions in relation to the identification of the caseload to be managed, the development of self and staff including acting as a mentor for case managers undergoing training and development, acting as a role model across services and organisations, development of policies and procedures for the service and of course act as a caseload manager. This is a broad set of leadership functions but each of them requires all the skills and behaviours previously outlined in this chapter. The need to facilitate clinicians' use of their knowledge and understanding to develop innovative ways to improve the systems for care has been a plea from a number of sources over the years [19].

A recent report from the National Nursing Research Unit in King's College London [20] clearly outlines the importance of practitioners as partners and leaders at the heart of health care. Practitioners as leaders continually challenge and improve care quality – they are ambitious for care particularly in relation to the role of nurses, they are confident innovators, they co-ordinate resources and skills to enable high-quality care and they supervise, monitor and teach carers, patients and other staff as appropriate to need. A vision of practitioners who continually champion care quality and use their voice in and across organisations to influence both policy and clinical practice is outlined and is very much in line with the expectations within all current national policies. This report supports the work on self-care and management in relation to the idea of practitioner and patient relationship as a partnership that enables increasing choice and self-determination for patients and the promotion of individualised patient-centred care. This concept of coproduction of care with practitioners providing leadership to enable this to occur across the NHS, local authorities and other agencies continues to gain momentum and credibility.

Leadership is in every role

The recent workforce report [21] also supports this concept of the practitioner as a partner and a leader. This report outlines the expectation that every practitioner will develop to offer leadership as appropriate to their skill level. The report also outlines, as already discussed, the variety of leadership positions in across teams, services and organisations that practitioners may wish to develop into, and it clearly defines the need for practitioners to 'step up and work with leaders' to enable changes in system for the benefit of patients. The balance of leadership and clinical work in roles will be dependent on the role but they are required to demonstrate leadership by keeping practice up to date and thereby delivering the best care for patients. The report contains a commitment by the Department of Health to work with professional bodies and regulators to ensure that these essential core skills (practitioner, partner and leader) are developed via education.

It is hoped that this work on essential core skills will lead to the inclusion in all training curricula teaching in relation to leadership skills. This will include a focus on leadership development for all junior doctors in postgraduate medical training and the introduction of a set of new standards in leadership, which can underpin leadership development programmes. The role of nurses as leaders who ensure the quality of care is a clear function and its importance is outlined in this report. The quality agenda in the NHS and its specific focus on safety, effectiveness and compassion will be supported through the membership on the National Quality Board of Chief Nursing Officer. This board will provide strategic oversight and leadership in relation to clinical priority setting and to approve the new quality measurement framework. The Department of Health is focused on the development of leadership abilities through the development of what are described as comprehensive continuing development programmes for nurses to equip them with the skills they will need to lead the quality charge through measurement, understanding and improvement. It is clear that the view is of nurse leaders within organisations demonstrating that they are not just leading but driving the quality agenda through acceptance of accountability for quality, which is measured through metrics. There has always been an understanding of the central role of leadership in the delivery of quality. Effective leadership is therefore essential to the delivery of the objectives of quality [22] and the current policy drivers and guidance clearly outline what the expectation is for leadership in the NHS, and quality clearly defines the expectation on delivery of this leadership.

Advanced practice

The concept of advanced practice is not a new one, particularly, in nursing, the Nursing and Midwifery Council (NMC) [23] along with a number of other professional bodies has defined advanced practice. In general, advanced practice can be defined as the ability of a practitioner to work or show skills that are well above the baseline expected competency for the profession.

The NMC defines advanced practice as

A registered nurse who has command of an expert knowledge base and clinical competence, is able to make complex decisions using expert clinical judgement, is an essential member of an interdependent health care team and whose role is determined by the context in which s/he practises.

Advanced nurse practitioners are highly experienced, knowledgeable and educated members of the care team who are able to diagnose and treat your health care needs or refer you to an appropriate specialist if needed.

NMC (2005)

Historically advanced roles in nursing had developed in a rather ad hoc way with a variation in training and competency definitions. The need to ensure that an advanced practitioner is fit for purpose has generated much debate across the professions, particularly as many advanced roles have developed in ways that mean the practitioner may be delivering an intervention usually carried out by another professional, for example diagnostics in primary care, prescribing, management of minor ailments in walk-in centre and accident and emergency environments, nurse and therapy consultant roles and roles such as physicians' assistants in the United States. Once practitioners develop skills and expertise outside the 'normal' for their profession there are debates in relation to appropriateness, professional protectionism and of course the important issue of patient safety.

A key problem in recent years in relation to advanced roles has been the paucity of information on how practitioners have developed competence and been prepared for these roles. In many areas, this preparation has been 'on the job' and while this may well be effective, it does not provide the level of confidence in relation to knowledge and skills levels held, which is required to ensure patient safety and confidence in the system. Until fairly recently, titles within nurse, particularly like nurse practitioner, nurse clinician and advanced practitioner, were available for use by almost any nurse. The use of these titles was confusing and it was not clear to patients what the titles meant with regard to competency levels or the ability of the practitioner. The NMC has now clearly defined the competency of an advanced practitioner and is supporting a process to ensure that practitioners who are employed in these roles are appropriately trained and competent. The NMC clearly states that only nurses who have achieved the competencies set out by the registration body can call themselves an advanced practitioner. The title is now protected through its definition as a registerable qualification on the professional council's register. This professional requirement includes a process for practitioners who may feel they have the skills and competence to meet the standards set to complete a process that enables the professional body to assess that they have achieved the required competence via education or experiential learning.

Prescribing

The ability to prescribe was once the remit of medical and dental practitioners in the main; however, the recent legislative changes have enabled a range of practitioners to join the family of prescribers. For prescribing by non medical practitioners (nurses, pharmacists and therapists), the NHS has been very clear regarding the standards of competence and educational preparation required to ensure safe practice [24]. All the professional bodies have published education standards for prescribing and the NMC and the National Prescribing Centre have published professional standards for prescribing with which practitioners are expected to comply [25,26]. The Royal Pharmaceutical Society of Great Britain and other professional bodies have also outlined professional standards for training and education in relation to prescribing.

Advanced practice in long-term conditions

In relation to the management of long-term conditions, the educational frame-work clearly outlines the requirements of practitioners as they relate to advanced practice [18]. These advanced practitioner competencies are in the main focused on the nursing role in case management, in particular that of the community matron. This advanced role is seen as one in which the nurse will utilise higher level examination and diagnostic skills supported by prescribing to enable the management of the clinical condition as outlined in the NMC definition of advanced practice. The ability to assess the medical condition of the patient by recognising changes in the disease process and to manage these appropriately is a key function in improving outcomes for those highly complex patients who are within the top 2–3% of the population with long-term conditions, often described as high-intensity users.

The NMC defines advanced practitioner as highly skilled nurses who can

- carry out physical examinations;
- use their expert knowledge and clinical judgement to decide whether to refer patients for investigations and make diagnoses;
- decide on and carry out treatment, including the prescribing of medicines, or refer patients to an appropriate specialist;
- use their extensive practice experience to plan and provide skilled and competent care to meet patients' health and social care needs, involving other members of the healthcare team as appropriate;
- ensure the provision of continuity of care including follow-up visits;
- assess and evaluate, with patients, the effectiveness of the treatment and care provided and make changes as needed;
- work independently, although often as part of a healthcare team that they will lead; and
- as a leader of the team, make sure that each patient's treatment and care is based on best practice.

This definition provides an excellent description of the requirements for community matrons in relation to managing long-term conditions. These requirements form the foundation on which educational programmes have been developed and are being delivered successfully across the NHS. Although there is currently little evidence in the UK context that advanced clinical skills contribute hugely to the success of case management programmes [27], the advanced practitioner skills do appear effective in enabling ongoing effective management of diseases and the continuity of care for patients.

As these patients require highly competent and confident practitioners who can manage their disease processes effectively through the whole episode of care, while at all times being mindful of the boundaries of their competency, it is helpful for practitioners to have a defined set of competence and skill they need to develop and are assessed against. It is in this important area of understanding boundaries and 'knowing what they do not know' that advanced practitioners are gradually developing their confidence as they through the partnerships and collaborations developed with medical and other specialist colleagues outline these boundaries and agree the processes for accessing support and review that are essential for the safety of these highly complex patients. These partnerships are the foundation of care delivery for these patients as the efficacy of services is dependent on the collaboration and partnerships that are developed across all care sectors not just with medical and other highly specialist services.

The ability to assess the clinical condition, to support the patient and carer, to understand how the disease progresses, to recognise deteriorations or changes in the condition and to plan and then implement early interventions for these changes does require a higher level of advanced clinical skills in the practitioner to deliver. The effectiveness of proactive management is dependant on a high level of clinical understanding of the disease process and what can be expected as the disease process. The ability to support the patient and carer to make decisions relating to how their health is managed in the longer term requires these advanced practitioner skills. Although advanced practice is not the only important skill for the management of long-term conditions, it is one of the skill sets that can add value to the process and can enable effective risk assessment of the clinical condition, which ensure patient safety.

Conclusions

Leadership and advanced practice are highly important in the modernised NHS and could be seen as fundamental to delivering effective management of long-term conditions. There is no debate that both of these are useful skills, which are required in the practitioners involved in managing high-intensity users through active case management, but it is also clear that these skills will provide added value to services if practitioners are able to develop them.

High-performing leaders are of course essential at all levels in the NHS and across all partner organisations. There is no doubt that organisations that have high-performing leaders from their clinical teams up to board are the organisations that will deliver the modernised services expected in all current health and social care policies. Those organisations that are quick to implement and bravely innovate, through excellent models of leadership, are the organisations that are most able to 'live' in the complex and changing environment of health and social care. There is also no doubt that an organisation that encourages and enables devolved leadership will be an organisation that is responsive and provides flexible models of service delivery. Effective leaders focus on interactions across organisations and environments. It is also clear that excellence in leadership is required in clinical teams to enable the quality and safety agenda to be delivered. Both clinical and nonclinical staff require leaders who facilitate self-direction and self-control not just management; therefore, effective leaders are clearly those who can facilitate and develop the skills of staff, providing the direction of travel and the support to allow staff to reach the end goal. Effective leaders will also share information and knowledge to fill any gaps in knowledge and understanding that become apparent in teams and staff as knowledge and information appropriately shared facilitates involvement and enables delivery.

Effective leaders must be able to engage all stakeholders in the development of a shared vision, ensuring that there is partnership in development and delivery, accountability is clearly outlined and agreed, a sense of ownership for the vision and strategy is fostered and there is equity in all processes involved in development of the vision or strategy and in their delivery. Good leaders accept and value diversity and create opportunities for learning and development. Highly performing leaders are self-aware and understand their function. They share leadership by giving authority away while ensuring accountability is clear and high performance is expected. Good leaders let the magic of innovation happen while ensuring that risks are mitigated. The sign of good leadership is the celebration of achievement of objectives being followed by time for a reflection on possible improvements or new ways of doing.

The abilities of practitioners to function as leaders must be developed as the NHS needs to prepare its leaders of the future and also because practitioners will more and more need to deliver leadership skills in the face of complex care systems and these functions are fundamental to ensuring the care delivered to patients is appropriate and effective. The requirement for nurses in particular to accept a role as leaders in relation to the quality of care in the NHS is ultimately a powerful tool to raise the profile of quality and advocacy of patient experience. The profile of the profession of nursing can only be raised by this leadership role in relation to quality. The NHS has high expectation of leadership – the Department of Health recently published 'Inspiring leaders: leadership for quality' [28] that outlines the journey the NHS, staff and patients are on to improve quality and the patient experience. The document published in support of the recent NHS Review outlines the talents required for the delivery of quality in services.

Although there is currently little definitive evidence at this time that advanced practitioner skills contribute to the effectiveness of case management in long-term conditions, the ability of practitioners to utilise these advanced skills to increase access, work with the patient to recognise changes in conditions and make plans to manage these changes in condition using early warning systems and planned interventions do appear to improve the experience for patients. The recognition of the need for a clear understanding of the competencies required in advanced practice provides for the public an assurance of the 'fitness to practice' of practitioners and the quality of the care they deliver. This process of defining the level and delivery expected of competence of practitioners is essential to enable the ongoing development of roles within the health and social care arena.

References

1. Obholzer (1997). *The Leader, The Unconscious and The Management of The Organisation.* New York ISBN 0-415-10206-5

2. Department of Health (2002). *National Health Service Leaderships Qualities Framework.* Accessed online on September 2008. http://www.dh.gov.uk/prod_consum_dh/groups/dh_digitalassets/@dh/@en/documents/digitalasset/dh_4083022.pdf

3. Department of Health (2008). *High Quality Care for All: NHS Next Stage Review Final Report.* http://www.dh.gov.uk/prod_consum_dh/groups/dh_digitalassets/@dh/@en/documents/digitalasset/dh_085828.pdf (accessed on October 2009).

4. World Class Commissioning, Department of Health (2008). *Commissioning Assurance Handbook.* http://www.dh.gov.uk/prod_consum_dh/groups/dh_digitalassets/@dh/@en/documents/digitalasset/dh_085141.pdf (accessed on October 2009).

5. Rothwell Douglas (2007). *The NHS North West Modernising Leadership Model.*

6. Cheshire & Merseyside Strategic Health Authority (2002). *Leading in Empowered Organisations: Report for Executive Nurses* (www.northwest.nhs.uk).

7. Carmel Hale (Facilitator) (June 2002). *RCN Clinical Leadership Programme Progress Report for the North West Region.* (www.northwest.nhs.uk)

8. Knowles D, Shakespeare G and Taylor J (1998). *Strategic Nurse Leadership Programme Report.* King's Fund. (www.kingsfund.co.uk)

9. Thomas P, McDonnell J, McCulloch J and Ferlie E (2002). *Facilitating Learning and Innovation in Primary Care Organisations.* Imperial College Business School, Brent Primary Care Trust. http://www.natpact.nhs.uk/uploads/fli.pdf (accessed on October 2009).

10. Nuffield Trust London (1999). *The Modern Values of Leadership and Management in the NHS.* http://www.bristol-inquiry.org.uk/images/sem4/0002/sem40002%20(0005-0021).pdf (accessed on October 2009).

11. Bate P (1994). *Organisational Culture and Leadership.* Oxford: Butterworth Heinemann.

12. Goleman D (1996). *Emotional Intelligence: Why It Can Matter More than IQ.* London: Bloomsbury Publishing.

13. Kitson A (2000). *Leadership Change and Learning from Experience.* Position Paper. Royal College of Nursing. http://www.rcn.org.uk/__data/assets/pdf_file/0009/78651/002524.pdf (accessed on October 2009).

14. Department of Health (2006). *Modernising Nursing Careers: Setting the Direction.* http://www.dh.gov.uk/prod_consum_dh/groups/dh_digitalassets/@dh/@en/documents/digitalasset/dh_4138757.pdf (accessed on October 2009).

15. Sefton Health Authority (1997). *Developing a Nursing Model for Effective Nursing Management and Professional Leadership.* (www.sefton.nhs.uk)

16. Modernisation Agency (2004). *Managing Long Term Conditions: A Self-Assessment Tool.* http://www.natpact.nhs.uk/cms/358.php#tools&templates (accessed on October 2009).

17. *An Examination of the Experience of Programme and Clinical Leads: Summary Report.* Evercare Programme 2004. http://www.natpact.nhs.uk/uploads/2005_Feb/Evercare_evaluation_interim_report.pdf

18. Department of Health (2006). *Caring for People with Long Term Conditions: An Educational Framework for Community Matrons and Case Managers.* http://www.dh.gov.uk/prod_consum_dh/groups/dh_digitalassets/@dh/@en/documents/digitalasset/dh_4118102.pdf (accessed on October 2009).

19. Royal College of General Practitioners and NHS Alliance (2004). *Clinicians, Services and Commissioning in Chronic Disease Management in the NHS. The Need for Co-ordinated Management Programmes.* http://www.rcgp.org.uk/PDF/Corp_chronic_disease_nhs.pdf (accessed on October 2009).

20. Maben J and Griffiths P (2008). *Nurses in Society: Starting the Debate.* National Nursing Research Unit, King's College London.

21. Department of Health (2008). *A High Quality Workforce: NHS Next Stage Review.* http://www.dh.gov.uk/prod_consum_dh/groups/dh_digitalassets/@dh/@en/documents/digitalasset/dh_085841.pdf (accessed on October 2009).

22. Wilson DC (1992). *A Strategy of Change: Programmed Approaches to Organisational Change*. Routledge. ISBN-13:978-1-86152-383-9 Cornwall
23. Nursing and Midwifery Council (2005). *Implementation of a Framework for the Standards of Post Registration Nursing*. http://www.nmc-uk.org/aArticle.aspx?ArticleID=82 (accessed on October 2009).
24. Department of Health (2002). *Extending Independent Nurse Prescribing with the NHS in England*. http://www.dh.gov.uk/prod_consum_dh/groups/dh_digitalassets/@dh/@en/documents/digitalasset/dh_4072177.pdf (accessed on October 2009).
25. Nursing and Midwifery Council (2007). *Standards for Proficiency for Nurse and Midwife Prescribing*. http://www.nmc-uk.org/aDisplayDocument.aspx?DocumentID=1645 (accessed on October 2009).
26. National Prescribing Centre (2003). *Maintaining Competency in Prescribing: An Outline Framework for Pharmacist Supplementary Prescribers*. http://www.npc.co.uk/prescribers/resources/competency_framework_oct_2006.pdf and http://www.npc.co.uk/prescribers/resources/nurse_update_framework.pdf (accessed on October 2009).
27. Association of Greater Manchester Primary Care Trusts (2005). *Implementing Active Case Management*. http://www.agmpcts.nhs.uk/news/
28. Department of Health (2008). *Inspiring Leaders: Leadership for Quality. Guidance for NHS Talent and Leadership Plans*. http://www.dh.gov.uk/prod_consum_dh/groups/dh_digitalassets/documents/digitalasset/dh_093407.pdf (accessed on October 2009).

Chapter 9
Self-Care and Patient Outcomes

Introduction

Historically, the organisation of services in the National Health Service (NHS) has relied on the passive nature of patients. Almost all the recent and current policy drivers for the NHS in recent years have focused on the ability of services to deliver and to ensure the delivery of improved capacity and capability for self-care and of improved outcomes, particularly patient-reported outcomes [1]. As early as 2000, the NHS Plan [2] outlined the need for services to become a resource for people to use routinely to enable them to look after themselves. It is clear that the direction of travel for the NHS and other services is to ensure that all services deliver interventions that focus on meeting the identified needs of patients and carers and of course provide added value to the service user. Self-care as described in this chapter is one of the building blocks for person-centred health care and of course case management of long-term conditions. In 2002 the Wanless review [3] supported the push for self-care and engagement in health by identifying the need for individuals to take responsibility for their own health, in what he describes as the 'fully engaged scenario', a policy that has been further developed within the NHS as will be shown later in this chapter. This policy of self-responsibility, care and management has been absolutely embedded in the NHS through the Choosing Health agenda [4].

What is self-care?

Self-care can be seen as part of every persons' daily life. There is a wide spectrum of self-care that ranges from total self-care and full independence (washing and dressing yourself) to 100% professional care (intensive care or surgery) and total dependence. The drive to develop and enable the abilities for self-care in patients with long-term conditions and in relation to their general health issues is, as outlined earlier, an underlying principle across all health policies. The NHS since its implementation has had an aim of provision of free health care for all at the point of need, this alongside the gradual development of healthcare interventions and professionals as experts in health has led to a loss of 'ownership' and responsibility for personal health in some ways. The 'pill for every ill' view is now thought to be not just as detrimental to health (impact of extensive antibiotic prescribing) but also having a negative impact on the ability of people to be 'in control' of their own destiny. This lack of control is both frustrating and dangerous as it denies a person the rights of self-determination.

Throughout NHS and social care policy therefore a central thread is now self-care, which enables the personal responsibility, personal choice and self-determination. This push towards individualised care is expected to promote and enable independence, though for those with long-term conditions this may need to be supported with community infrastructure. The publication of the NHS Constitution in 2009 [5], following the consultation on the format published in late 2008, is the latest in the long line of documents that try to clarify and agree on not only the expectation patients should have of the NHS but also the expectation the NHS will have of them with personal responsibility for health and self-care being the key aspects. Some of these discussions on personal responsibility relate to improving health behaviours and lifestyles to reduce the potential risk of development of chronic disease by reduction in obesity and smoking and increasing physical exercise rates across communities. It is clear that the ability to self-care, particularly in relation to managing their own health, for those who suffer long-term conditions is dependent on education and development of knowledge. This would include how much they know in relation to their condition(s), the ways in which the condition(s) progresses and how they can 'do something' personally to maintain their own health and work towards better health behaviours and lifestyle. It is clear that this understanding alongside excellent standards of disease management should slow the progress of diseases and therefore improve the health outcomes and reduce negative impacts.

Department of Health guidance [6] on developing and promoting self-care clearly outlines the potential impact effective self-care can have on utilisation of resources in the NHS. Evidence from the guidance explains that self-care could

- reduce visits to general practitioners (GPs) by up to 40%;
- reduce visits to outpatients by up to 17%;
- reduce accident and emergency (A&E) visits by up to 50%; and
- reduce the drugs bill.

The impacts for patients as described by the Department of Health are as follows:

- Experience better health and well-being;
- Improved medicines concordance;
- Prevent need for emergency health and social services;
- Maintain independence in their own home;
- Increased confidence and sense of control;
- Improved mental health and reduction in levels of depression.

These claims are the underpinning evidence for the development of NHS programmes such as Expert Patient Programme (EPP) [7], the ongoing development of disease-related education and self-management programmes and the push to train all frontline staff in the principles of self-care.

Since the Department of Health identified the requirement to improve the management of long-term conditions as one of its top priorities, the push to increase self-care abilities has been a thread through the centre of all service plans. It has been described that a patient with diabetes will receive on average 3 hours of contact with professionals per year and they personally provide their own care for the remaining 8757 hours in the year [7]. This information therefore makes it clear that the professionals need to ensure that patients can develop the skills they need to maintain their own health. If a patient has the ability to self-care, they are more able to make choices and decisions that will in the longer term improve their health outcome. It is also clear that self-care works for both patients and staff. Professor Chris Ham in the foreword to *Promoting Optimal Self Care* [8] explains very clearly that there is evidence that self-care is effective in improving the quality of peoples' lives and it promotes the appropriate use of services.

The majority of people with long-term conditions would wish to remain independent and carry on with their lives in a way that is appropriate for them. As outlined earlier, the majority of care delivered to people with long-term conditions is carried out away from the health service – the patients do this care themselves or are supported by carers, family and friends. The problem with this self-care is that it is sometimes not optimal and therefore does not deliver the outcomes expected. *Promoting Optimal Self Care* [8] therefore describes the need to design clinical interventions and pathways with the aim of promoting self-care.

There are currently two terms in use, 'self-care' and 'self-management', which are at times used interchangeably, and in an attempt to clarify the process the Department of Health has defined each of these terms.

Self-care is 'about individuals taking responsibility for their own health and well-being. This includes: staying fit and healthy, both physically and mentally; taking action to prevent illness and accidents; and the better use of medicines and treatment of minor ailments', Department of Health (2001) (quoted in Ref. [8]).

Self-management is defined as

> The individual's ability to manage the symptoms, treatment, physical and psychosocial consequences and lifestyle changes inherent with living with a long term disorder.
>
> Department of Health (2001) (quoted in Ref. [8])

Based on these definitions, self-management is therefore a part of self-care.

Another definition provided by the Department of Health for self-care is

> ... the actions people take for themselves, their children and their families to stay fit and maintain good physical and mental health: meet social and psychological needs, prevent illness or accidents; care for minor ailments and long term conditions; maintain health and well being after acute illness or discharge from hospital.
>
> Department of Health [9]

There is a complex relationship between the severity of a disease and the quality of life for a patient, the understanding of which is still being developed, but we know that in relation to long-term conditions a number of key issues determine the quality of life. These range from the ability to communicate with professionals and manage their medication to personal adjustments and family dynamics in relation to their disease. The key though is that the patients understand the disease and its progress and impact as only then can they control their life in any meaningful way.

Self-care and practitioners

The 'Common core principles to support self care' from Skills for Care [10] provides a challenge to commissioners, practitioners and service providers to reflect and review how they commission and deliver personalised services that promote independence and choice. This document clearly outlines for practitioners the need for two-way communication, negotiation and partnership in decision making. The process of developing self-care abilities is not about professionals totally handing over responsibility but is about enabling the patient to contribute to planning and management process to achieve the best possible outcome for the patient. This entails giving some element of control and responsibility for their own health to people working in partnership and collaboration with the professionals and care agencies. This sharing on responsibility can only succeed if the patient understands the disease(s) and is confident in that understanding. This process of sharing responsibility is seen as placing the patient at the centre of the planning process and underpins the personalisation of care agenda outlined in 'Our Health, Our Care, Our Say' [11] and a wide range of other NHS and social care policies.

'Putting people first' [12] outlines the expectation for adult social services and of course the staff that people irrespective of illness or disability will be supported to

- Live independently;
- Stay healthy and recover quickly from illness;
- Exercise maximum control over their own life and where appropriate to lives of their family members;
- Sustain the family unit avoiding the need for children to take on inappropriate caring roles;
- Participate as active and equal citizens, both economically and socially;
- Have the best possible quality of life, irrespective of illness or disability;
- Retain the maximum dignity and respect.

These expectations are clearly matched to those with all NHS guidance and policy in relation to self-care, choice and independence.

It is important to remember that all NHS and social care roles will have within their job description something that relates to enabling and empowering patients for independence and choice. Case management professionals in particular, across the NHS and social care, are heavily involved in the promotion of self-care/management. In fact from a patient's perspective, their key function is to enable independence and improved outcomes. The competencies that all these roles utilise to enable the delivery of this function should be clearly outlined within their job description, and for case manager role they should be specifically outlined within the educational requirements.

Systems for self-care

The Department of Health has outlined some key points in the patients' journey through care [6] in which self-care can be delivered and supported and has identified the tools that can be utilised for these key points to facilitate effective self-care. It is clear from Department of Health guidance that the systems in place for promoting self-care for people with long-term conditions need to provide

- Information that is both understandable and accessible;
- Training so that patients can recognise and monitor their own symptoms;
- Appropriate support to enable the development of confidence and skills;
- Information and education, in an understandable format, relating to medicines, their use and importance, in managing the disease process.

A self-care/management system that provides these will probably then provide for patients

- Diagnosis, treatment and access to services in a timely manner;
- Understandable information, which is of good quality;
- Ongoing community-based care;
- Appropriate sharing of information between professionals, which is effective and timely;
- Co-ordinated and consistent services.

Expert Patient Programme

The EPP [7] provides for patients with long-term conditions self-care skills and training. The programme provides to patients support in developing skills, confidence and competence to 'care for themselves' through an understanding of their condition, confidence in asking questions to professionals and an ability to cope with the pressures and changes a long-term condition places on their lives. The programme was implemented well in some areas but implementation across the NHS was patchy. The programme is now delivered under a national contract by a key provider who works with local organisations to provide the programme to patients identified locally. The EPP recognises that health professionals cannot empower a patient, but can with lay/peer support assist patients to develop the strategies and skills they need to become empowered. It is also clear from the advice in the EPP that ongoing support to maintain self-management/care skills is required as initial education does not last forever.

Effectiveness of self-care programmes

When the NICE Review [13] of the evidence base in relation to broad-based generic self-management programmes in the United Kingdom was completed, it highlighted the limited nature of evaluations of EPP. In the main, the support for the programme is based on research into programmes run outside the United Kingdom. There are of course differences between EPP and the self-management programmes developed in other countries, not the least of which is the requirement for patients with specific conditions to be referred following confirmed diagnosis by physician, whereas the EPP programme allows self-referral of people who identify that they have a chronic condition. So any person who wishes to sign up for a course may do so, which may have an impact on the outcomes of the programme. An internal evaluation of EPP by the Department of Health indicates some very positive results with reduction in GP contact by 7%, in outpatient visits by 10% and in accident and emergency attendances by 16% and with increases in health information uptake by 34% and in improved consultations by 33%. These findings are encouraging but a broader based review is required.

All initial pilots of EPP identified some barriers to implementation. It is clear from these findings that programmes within primary care trusts (PCTs) in urban areas and who appoint a lead administrator are more successful. The success is also assisted by raising awareness and robust recruitment via the local press or other media approaches and by networking PCTs to deliver.

There are a number of factors that will contribute to patients' ability to self-care and make appropriate decisions to change their behaviour to promote healthy choices. These factors are

- history and life experience;
- existing knowledge;
- values and beliefs;
- cultural background;
- literacy and cognitive ability;
- confidence, self-esteem and self-efficacy;
- perceived control;
- availability of real, personalised choice;
- availability of information and the form in which the information is presented;
- availability of useful tools and equipment;
- evidence on benefits of self-care support
- encouragement by practitioners.

It is therefore important that all models of support to self-care take cognisance of these factors for individuals as one size will not fit all.

The delivery of education and advice focused in a disease-specific way is highly important and though the EPP does provide an overview of some disease areas, it cannot by definition provide the level of knowledge and understanding in each specific disease areas that would be required for the process to be totally effective. A number of disease-specific interest groups have developed information and educational programmes for their area that are effective in enabling the patient to understand the progress of their disease and how they can influence this.

The Institute for Healthcare Improvement [13] clearly defines what it sees as essential areas of understanding to enable patients to become effective managers of their own health. The Institute's reviews of service improvement show that in order to ensure patients can manage their own health they must have a basic understanding of their disease, ongoing support from networks (professional teams, family and community) and support to enable them to build the skills and confidence to self-manage (knowing when and why to access assistance). This process should also include education of patients about the guidelines for the management of their disease through patient-friendly information (handouts and information posted in clinics) and support for providers to ensure messages are delivered in a clear and equitable way. It is also clear from all the evidences that there is a need to ensure patients are empowered through collaboration in goal setting and involvement in decision making.

The Institute for Healthcare Improvement [14] has also provided advice in relation to evidence of effectiveness of self-management tools and information. This advises professionals to review with their team all materials to ensure all are using the information consistently and the information is understood and credible in the team, to test materials with patients and ask for feedback on appropriateness and to use the feedback to improve the materials in use. Further advice is available relating to the need to ensure information is appropriate and is available to a broad range of needs and of course formats (languages and literacy levels) and to ensure that the information can be delivered to all in an equitable and appropriate way. The need to ensure information is shared with a wide range of colleagues (pharmacies and community groups) is also highly important and effective in ensuring information gets to those who need it.

Promoting self-care: staff role

The seven principles expected from staff involved in developing self-care outlined in the 'Common core principles to support self care' are as follows:

- Ensure individuals are able to make informed choices to manage their self-care needs;
- Communicate effectively to enable individuals to assess their needs, and develop and gain confidence to self-care;

- Support and enable individuals to access appropriate information to manage self-care needs;
- Support individuals to use technology to support self-care;
- Advise individuals how to access support networks and participate in planning, development and evaluations of services;
- Support and enable risk management and risk taking to maximise choice and independence.

These principles are described as competencies that include expected behaviours and knowledge that underpins these behaviours. The carers involved in the development process for these principles felt that they would provide a useful set of tools for staff and that they were evidence of a positive drive for improvement in services. It is clear that the value base that underpins self-care is one of supporting and empowering, changing the focus of power within the relationship between professionals and service users. This can be seen as a challenge for professionals and will require supervision, appraisal and development to make sure they become embedded in services. The responsibility to ensure standards of care in services rests with leaders and managers of services and they must ensure that services are delivered in a way that achieves the aim of personalisation, focusing on dignity, respect, choice and control for patients. To ensure that services can support and facilitate self-care/management, it is clearly important that professionals are appropriately educated and trained. Services should also ensure that shared decision making can be supported through the further development of the decision support software and other initiatives being trailed across the NHS.

Self-care: models

Patients need to make adjustments to how they live their lives when they are diagnosed with a long-term condition and it is clear from the literature review completed by the King's Fund [15] that there are a number of things that shape how people respond and adjust. However, it is clear that immediate behaviour change and compliance with medication advice may not be delivered by structured self-management education as the social, psychological and emotional feelings of the patient may prevent an immediate positive response. It is also clear that a person's ability to self-care will change over time; it may increase or decrease. A review of the literature highlights that the ability of a patient to participate in self-management is heavily influenced by length of time since diagnosis, severity of disease, age, social support, stage of their life and level of education. Reviews of successful programme have in the past reported that participators in self-management programmes tend to be women, younger, middle class and better educated [16]. For some patients it may still be their view that they prefer to do what the doctor decides. So those involved in managing patients with long-term conditions need to be mindful that every patient's response will be unique.

The historical approach to changing health behaviours is one of negative commands. We now know that it is vital to recognise that pleasure is derived from some of the unhealthy habits and we need to utilise different approaches to make positive health behaviours the norm. It is known that information alone does not change behaviour, to be successful a broad range of interventions are required and different areas of poor health behaviour may require different approaches. The professionals do provide some help to patients in this area, but they alone cannot deliver all the support required for change, other organisations are also important (i.e. employer's and local authorities).

Currently patients can access health care in a wide variety of ways, from 999 for emergencies to attendance at a screening clinic. The ability of the public to make appropriate use of the NHS is encouraged via the NHS Constitution [5], which outlines the broad rights and responsibilities of patients who utilise NHS services. It is sometimes argued that the NHS should make patients aware of the cost if they are to make more appropriate use of its resources; this approach is based on an assumption that patients abuse or overuse services. Offering patients' choice of appointments based on informed choices can also reduce waste of services.

The National Primary Care Research and Development Centre has produced 'The WISE approach to self-management' [17], which outlines the ways in which clinicians can engage patients in a shared approach to self-management. This approach outlines the strategy and methods in relation to the patient, the professional and the structure. In the WISE model the strategy for the patient is to improve information, and this is done by working with the patients to develop relevant and accessible information, which uses both lay and traditional evidence bases for knowledge. For the professional the strategy is to change the response, promoting flexibility to the way the professional acts to enable a patient-centred approach and negotiate for self-management plans with the patient. The structure requires a strategy that improves access to services through changes to access arrangements using professional and patient contacts as a way of complimenting processes to maximise effectiveness of management of diseases and allowing the patient to self-refer based on a personal evaluation of need for advice. Salford NHS Hospitals Trust has used this approach very effectively, and work reviewing possible impact in primary care is progressing.

The 'Working in Partnership Programme' has developed the 'Self Care for Primary Care Professionals Project' [18] that Central Cheshire Primary Care Trust has been implementing. The scheme defines what self-care is and the actions that may be taken to promote self-care including a process known as the cycle of self-care. The aims of the project are to provide multidisciplinary training package for teams to develop self-care knowledge and skills, implement an integrated approach to patient- and professional-led model of self-care, assist in the development of a self-care strategy for the organisations and provide access to the appropriate evidence base and best practice. The training package provided gives an overview of the context and evidence base for self-care, up to date information in relation to management of minor ailments together with advice on development of joint guidelines for conditions to be self-managed and advice on how the practice can ensure consistent messages across the team.

Primary Care Contracting produced in 2007 [19] an enhanced service framework for supporting self-care in primary care. This framework provides to commissioners and providers a service outline with clear objectives and outcomes. It also provides clear guidance on provision, competence of staff, governance and information requirements. The framework aims to simplify for commissioners the process of procuring effective services and also to encourage primary care to deliver.

Self-care: the evidence base

The evidence base for lay-led self-management has been reviewed by National Institute for Health and Clinical Excellence [13]. This approach to providing self-care advice is aimed at the 70–80% of the population with long-term conditions who require the lower levels of healthcare support and intervention. The review identified clearly that managing long-term conditions is not simply a health issue but requires a broad range of social support to manage the social and psychological impact of chronic conditions.

The NICE Review reviewed a fairly broad body of research to identify how lay people manage self-care and live a normal life. The review findings highlight from research the following three key types of 'work' that lay people with chronic disease do:

- Illness work (managing symptoms and diagnostic-related work);
- Everyday life (doing the daily tasks);
- Biographical work (reforming the life of the patient).

This thorough review of evidence to date [20] highlights some key implications for self-management of chronic conditions. The key concepts from seven of the studies reviewed described how patients balanced the need to be in control and feel well against the disorder they feel during episodes of ill-health; this has a major impact on the patients' abilities in relation to self-care. The literature reviewed also clearly confirmed that though the recent policy initiatives apparently describe a situation in which there is little or no self-management, it is actually very well established, and in fact quite sophisticated within communities.

This review also reaffirmed the impact of social factors on patient's ability to self-manage, in particular the issues of age and social class are described as highly important when seeking to improve abilities to self-manage as they will clearly affect the processes utilised. The ability of patients to maintain a social identity is a very *delicate balance* and the ability of a patient to maintain viable social roles and therefore identity is extremely important.

This review also confirmed very clearly that while there are some common problems that can be identified among those with chronic diseases, the circumstances of the individual will have a huge effect. There is therefore no uniformity in the problems experienced and thus there is no 'one size fits all' response. The reviewer also devoted some time to identify the practical problems in relation to implementation of programmes and highlighted quality of leadership, adequate infrastructure including sufficient trainers and lay leaders, the presence of commitment and passion and a successful recruitment processes. Recruitment is often seen as a major problem in the generic programmes and if disease-specific programmes are available locally.

The way patients 'live' within their community with a chronic disease is very different to the way the medical model of life progresses, and it is clear that patients can be highly adaptable, challenging the assumptions of professionals about what and how their lives can be 'improved'. Lay-led self-management processes are very different from the 'traditional' approaches to self-management provided through health care and professionals. Lay-led self-management models are routed in the idea that the patient requires motivation, a sense of self-confidence and self-efficacy when dealing with the disease and its impacts. The conclusion of this review is that health care must base all interventions and responses on robust assessment of the needs of patients with long-term conditions and that health care should beware of a focus on empirical insights and externally mediated management approaches.

Early lay-led self-management programmes tended to be disease specific and based on a holistic care model focusing on specific outcomes relating directly to the disease [21], for example asthma programme focusing on peak flow measures and arthritis programmes focusing on pain and function. In the United States during 1990s, Kaiser Permanente developed a Chronic Disease Management Program [22], providing generic self-management advice based on the assumptions that patients with chronic conditions have similar self-management problems and tasks to complete, that patients can learn to take responsibility for their own day-to-day management and that confident, knowledgeable patients who can manage themselves will utilise less healthcare resource. The programme was offered over seven sessions, which included a range of health-related issues including problem solving, improved health behaviours, medication concordance and managing emotional impacts of disease. The ongoing evaluation of this programme identified some positive benefits in relation to maintenance of independence despite worsening levels of disability, but there was little evidence of major improvement in other expected areas, for example access to services. Unfortunately, the findings of some of the early evaluations [23] completed of self-management programmes in the United Kingdom have not reported the expected levels of improvement, with only small to moderate impacts across the areas.

All self-management programmes, generic or disease-specific, have the similar key aims and expected outcomes, and though the delivery formats may differ slightly, all aim to empower and enable the patient and their carers. Almost every programme relies on self-selection/recruitment to some extent, which could impact the types of patients who join. It is clear in the NICE Review [20] that many of the participants in programmes are women and that the level of education of participants tends to be fairly high. The educational level of participants can have a major impact on the effectiveness of the programmes, with patients with higher educational levels having better outcomes. It is also clear that despite the higher levels of disease in 'underprivileged' groups, they are the least likely to access self-management programmes, which could mean that the overall impact of programmes will be heavily influenced by health inequalities.

Using information and technology for self-care

Information and how it is used is the key to enabling self-care/management – the requirement for professionals to share information and work with patients to consider the best way to manage their condition and any changes that may occur. Patients do occasionally not wish to be in control and in these circumstances the pressure on patients to engage in the process must be handled with great care.

The NHS White Paper [24] was committed to the introduction of information on prescription for all long-term health conditions. This paper proposed:

> To give all people with long term health and social care need and their carers an 'information prescription'. The information prescription will be given to people using services and their carers by health and social care professionals to signpost people to further information and advice to help them take care of their own condition.
>
> By 2008, we would expect everyone with a long term condition and/or long term need for support – and their carers – to routinely receive information about their condition and, where they can, to receive peer and other self care support through networks.
>
> Department of Health [24]

To aid the implementation of this programme, the department recruited 20 pilot sites to test the programme and provide evidence on effectiveness [25]. Many of the pilots worked in partnership arrangements with voluntary organisations and statutory agencies such as health and social care, and across a wide range of settings (acute, primary care and mental health). The programmes related to a broad range of conditions including Parkinson's disease, arthritis, cancer, sight loss and diabetes. This evaluation outlined the following five main parts to an information prescription:

- Information content: reliable and relevant sources;
- Directories
- Personalised process: information must be specific to the condition, the place and the point at which care has reached;

- Issuing: the importance of how an information prescription is created and provided to a patient;
- Access: how information is made available.

The evaluation was limited by delays in implementation in pilot areas, slightly lower uptake than expected and insufficient time to complete longer term impact studies. The evaluation did not use any randomisation or experimental design and this limits the robustness of the findings.

The pilot sites completed the following three main stages for the programme:

- Preparation: it enabled them to define information prescriptions for themselves and develop a local focus.
- Development: this included broader engagement with all quality assuring information, developing IT solutions and training of those who would disseminate information.
- Delivery: the pilots delivered the 'prescriptions' in differing ways dependent on nature of the user population and local pressures.

The pilots defined information prescriptions differently with some clearly being uncomfortable with the concept of 'prescribing' as this medicalised the process. But despite this issue most of the pilots developed a common set of principles to underpin development, which included involvement of users, carers and professionals. The need to engage widely patients, carers, professionals and other agencies to support the process was highly important to implementation. All pilot areas stressed the need for information to be 'quality assured' and many links to the processes utilised by partner agencies to support this process. IT solutions including websites where they were available assisted greatly in the success of pilots, but the sophistication of the IT systems available and the ability of the staff and users involved to utilise them was variable. Training was incredibly important as those involved in providing 'prescriptions' needed a level of knowledge to enable them to safely and effectively answer questions raised or understand when to refer for specialist advice. Delivery of prescription was done by a broad range of professionals, and in the main the models of delivery were influenced by

- How prescriptions could be personalised.
- How to ensure access to the most disadvantaged.

These issues were seen as important, but as would be expected, each of the pilots managed these in different ways. Personalisation of information as a key issue was managed by

- Mapping care pathways with users and carers to establish stages of care and the information needs;
- Using the pathways to develop templates to identify information a user needs and when;
- Developing structures scripts and prompts;
- Consulting users on their preferred method for receiving information;
- Ensuring the information prescriptions are easily accessible to all;

- Providing extra support to those who are disadvantaged or unable to access;
- Providing information at locations that are easy to access and at which users congregate, particularly those who are disadvantaged;
- Providing information through different processes: telephone etc.;
- Providing information in a variety of formats.

This evaluation reported some positive impacts and outcomes for patients. Seventy-three per cent of patients felt better able and more confident when asking questions relating to their condition, although the numbers were lower in those who described their health as poor (62%). Over half of the patients (52%) felt that the information provided improved their care; however, the figure was slightly lower in those aged under 65 (44%) and in people who got their prescriptions via primary care (42%). In the areas that chose to offer information via what are described as 'light touch' methods (access via self-dispensing and with limited personalisation and support), the rates were 45%. The rates for information prescriptions via acute care and for those in affluent areas were 62%. When asked about a feeling of being in control of what was happening to them and their condition, 66% had positive views, but there were marked variations – patients under 65 years reported only 55%; mental health patients, 57%; those who believed themselves to be in 'poorer health', 52%; and those in deprived areas, 52%.

Eighty-two per cent of carers who had seen or were aware of the information, when asked felt that the information provided was useful, but 35% were unaware of the information prescriptions despite being within pilot areas. The professionals involved in issuing information prescriptions reported being very or fairly satisfied with the process in their areas. The response result was noticeably lower in GPs and pratice nurses.

A key challenge for the pilots in relation to supporting patients with long-term conditions were the difficulties experienced in relation to the provision of high enough levels of support, particularly for those with higher levels of need and those who are disadvantaged. The other key challenge identified by the pilots was the problem of variation and inconsistencies in approaches, which might lead to some users not receiving information when they should.

The findings of this evaluation [26] clearly support the further development of the information prescription model and make recommendations on how the process can be made more effective for patients, carers and staff. These recommendations include the importance of full involvement in development (carers, patients, voluntary groups and all professional groups), ensuring that information prescriptions are delivered in a truly personalised way and that directories contain sufficient information for the patient to manage their condition and access services across health and social care. Other key recommendations are as follows:

- The development of templates for providing information nationally, and which can be refined and used locally;
- Development of a national directory of information storing accredited information using a national accreditation scheme to ensure quality;

- Local models must allow for the needs of disadvantaged or hard to reach groups;
- All areas of care (whole systems) approaches must be used in the development of programmes;
- Carers must be fully engaged and involved in the process to ensure full efficacy of the process;
- Staff must be supported to develop and embed the skills required to deliver information prescriptions appropriately and this should form part of the ongoing professional education and competency development processes.

In 2005 the Department of Health [27] had completed a review of 19 papers on technologies in use for either health behaviour modification (e.g. step-o-meters) or self-monitoring (e.g. glucose monitoring) in an attempt to understand the pros and cons of the use of technology. Although the report is not a systematic review, its findings do add to the debate and understanding relating to technology and its uses in self-care. The report is in the main very positive in its comments on many of the programmes in use. The authors commented that some of the cheapest and simplest devices showed considerable scope for improved health outcomes, and that the continuous monitoring devices at that time appeared to offer real opportunities. However, in the view of the authors, following are the main problems for technology:

- Control monitoring programmes require central support and this has hidden cost during implementation;
- Standards of devices are not always clear;
- Systems and devices do not work together;
- Lack of combined evaluation/joint research may limit the opportunities for effective implementation.

Some patients are supported with self-management via assistive technology such as distant testing, email for communication and advice and text messaging. It is clear from the report 'Engaging patients in their health' [20] that technology could be very useful in self-care and is currently significantly underdeveloped. Although patients may use the Internet to access information and this may have changed the nature of social relationships, the use of the Internet by health care is very limited. NHS Direct Online and NHS Choices are gradually being developed for patients to develop their own content. Technology could play a very effective role in identifying patients who might benefit from health interventions and has been used by some organisation to improve the management of patients at the lower level of the risk pyramid for long-term conditions. In the United States, Medalink is used effectively by families for searching a wide range of information in relation to diseases, symptoms and services. The people who access the system also want to store the information to create a resource of health knowledge for themselves. The problem with searching on the 'web' for information is that the information accessed will not always be of a high standard and probably not be of any use to the searcher.

There are existing technologies that health and social care could utilise to improve health, for example radio, digital television, DVDs, telephone and email, all could be used to deliver messages to a wide range of people. Some such as the telephone can deliver personalised messages, whereas the others could be used for broader messages. Although there are a range of technologies available, it is clear that the technical solutions must be needs-led not driven by the technology, and further evaluation of the effectiveness of self-monitoring and support is needed.

How do we engage patients in self-care?

It is clearly extremely important that professionals develop good relationships with patients to enable support to self-care/management. The relationship will be improved and made more effective if the patient feels that the professional has the ability to listen, understands the main concerns the patient has, allows the patient the time needed, can understand the impact of the disease on the patient and enables the patient to contribute to the planning of their care. Patients who are noncompliant are often a problem for professionals in managing long-term conditions, but this is often related to differing views between professionals and patients in relation to the explanations of care being based on clinical models that are not understood or not real for patients; it is therefore important that professionals are clear and understand the context of the patients' life. The United Kingdom is noted [20] as one of the worse performers in almost all indicators for engaging patients on their care. Fewer patients report involvement in treatments decisions and medication reviews or being given information about medication side effects. The patients also report less support relating to rehabilitation and recovery and worryingly less than one in five patients with a long-term condition report being given a self-management plan.

The provision of information to patients is one of the key ways to engage patients in their care. The information provided as outlined previously must be of good quality and sufficient in amounts to be effective. The patients should also be appropriately signposted to professionals and others who can provide advice and support in an effective and flexible way. Patients are aware that professionals' time is at a premium and that services are often pressured, but it remains clear that long-term conditions management needs time to deliver the support required to enable self-management/care.

One approach to successful engagement with the public is to move our focus from services users as patients to consumers; the concept of a patient can be seen as a passive role rather than as active in the process to do the things. A consumer is viewed as someone who makes use of services, obtains information and makes choices on the services they use. It is generally thought that when people act as consumers this changes the relationship between the user and the professional and can improve the quality and outcome of the care delivered. The changing expectations of patients are supporting this – although there will always be circumstances in which patients will wish professionals to make decisions for them, the patients with long-term conditions are rapidly increasing their expectation in relation to shared decision making and self-care [14].

If the NHS is to change and put the patient at the centre of care, then it needs to deliver case management and its predictive, preventive and participatory processes. The focus needs to be shifted to being customer-focused to maximise quality of life for patients and to enable more care to be delivered closer to home. Patients with chronic conditions access health care mainly when they have a problem, for the rest of their time they want to carry on with their lives. It may be that in the future the relationship with the NHS and caring service will be more ongoing to keep them as healthy as possible. The Department of Health [25] has identified that 82% of people with a long-term condition feel they take an active role in caring for it, but it is also clear from Department of Health data [6] that only 50% of medication prescribed is used after collection.

For the NHS to engage with people the messages must be constant and clear and where possible should be available across a broad range of media; the messages must be out in the system every day. It is also clear that for the process of engagement and self-care to be successful, it cannot be the responsibility of the NHS alone. The NHS needs to engage much more broadly groups such as the voluntary sector, social care and local communities to assist and support in the delivery of the self-care agenda. Engagement with patients is variable across services and the report from the King's Fund [20] highlighted that while the key source of information on health for most people is their GP, they see the GP on average twice a year, so the time available is probably less than 20 minutes. This report also discusses the impact of poor health behaviours learned and formed well in advance of any contact with professionals and the need to enable behaviour change to support people in the development of confidence and ability to self-manage and self-care. The report 'Public attitudes to self-care' [26] published in 2005 also highlights some concerning findings from patients which highlight that 44% of them felt that their GP did not encourage them to play an active role in the management of their long-term conditions.

Conclusions

The ability of patients to 'learn' to self-care is highly dependent on a number of issues, not least of which is their motivation to do something. Although professionals now understand that self-management is a good idea, we have historically disempowered patients from decision making, and the change of direction will take time to achieve. In fact it may be that we need to focus our effort on developing these self-care skills in people before they fall ill, as it is clear that health habits are formed long before people come into contact with the NHS. We therefore need to reflect on how as professionals we might utilise the models outlined in this chapter with the support of behaviour modification skills required to enable change to happen and be successful. Bandura noted that 'if the huge benefits of a few key lifestyle habits were put into a pill, it would be declared a spectacular breakthrough in the field of medicine' (quoted in Ref. [16]).

We understand that providing information on risks to health and what they should do rarely on its own is effective and for this reason many, if not all, of the programmes for self-care or self-management include or provide as an extra support process interventions to enable behaviour change programmes.

For behavioural change to be successful, it needs to turn an 'intention to change' into an action and it also requires that the behaviour change is maintained over time. The theories of behaviour change are well established [16] though not empirically supported. Behaviour change is reliant on the expectation of favourable outcomes and the patients feeling confident that they can perform the new behaviour. Long-term maintenance of behaviour change requires early recognition of lapses and management, so that they do not become permanent. The ability of patients to set goals for themselves and assess the achievements of these goals as part of a personalised plan is the key to enabling behaviour change and therefore self-care/management.

The major changes in health policy in recent years mean that it is clear that the NHS must now change its modus operandi from a sickness service into a service that promotes wellness in its broadest terms. Prevention of chronic disease that affects so much of the population is seen as a key priority and the NHS has a key role in helping the population to become healthier. Behavioural change whether in relation to prevention of chronic disease or self-management is hugely important. To enable change a person would need both motivation (a reason for action and an enthusiasm) and confidence (a belief in ones own ability to succeed). Some of the forms of intervention that promote confidence and motivation are

- peer modelling
- buddying
- group programmes
- assessment of an individual's readiness for change
- staged interventions
- motivational interviewing

The need to commission, develop and deliver programmes of this type is highlighted in reports from the King's Fund [28, 29]. It is clear from these reports that the ability to improve the health of the population relies on the implementation of behavioural change programmes, and their implementation will only happen if commissioners commission. The expectation on primary care trusts is that they will improve the health of their local population; therefore, public health programmes that support local people to stop smoking, be more active, eat a healthy diet, etc. must be central to their strategic commissioning plans. As all commissioning organisations have now produced their 5-year commissioning plans, which are expected to focus on reducing health inequalities and improving the general health of the population, the expectation is that programmes that promote healthy life choices will be at the centre of the activity by the NHS and its partner organisations including the third sector.

The personalised care agenda very clearly requires professionals and services to recognised and work with the patients as decision makers in their care; this describes the patient as a co-producer of health [16]. Eighty-seven per cent of patients with long-term conditions are keen to play a greater role in managing their disease. Although this desire varies across age, disease, educational status and of course the stage of a disease, it remains clear that professional assumptions about what patients want often are incorrect. There is a real need for professional attitudes to be changed and there is some evidence that this is happening, though this evidence is anecdotal rather than measured objectively. Although there is evidence that motivation and confidence are key in delivering successful behaviour change and through this the ability to self-manage/ care, there is no real evidence that says one approach is more effective than the other. But the challenges to delivery are now clear as are the processes that facilitate and improve the ability of services to reach patients and make some impact on their lives. The best approaches are those that are patient-orientated and help the patients live with their disease and do not just push information to the patients. The programmes must be interactive and using peers (those who are comfortable with self-management) to support and deliver the process does seem to make sense as it enables reality for patients. The training of staff in relation to self-management is also highly important; it is clear from the programmes outlined in this chapter that the most effective are those where professionals are taught not to 'lecture' but to discuss and enable. Also important to success is the need to let patient concerns lead the process and to take a slow but sure approach to behavioural change, thereby developing confidence in patients. These processes supported by agreed goals with patients (patients led), which are documented, and regular follow-up and appropriate support will enable the success of self-care processes. The initiatives and policies (EPP, technology, self-care programmes) reviewed in this chapter and of course guidance such as National Service Frameworks provide the frame on which organisations and professionals in partnerships with patients, carers and other agencies can deliver a self-care system that works.

As there are some risks inherent in processes supporting self-care, the professionals, patients and carers must develop the ability to consider fully and manage the risks, to enable and deliver the patient-led NHS services, which policymakers are pushing for. The provision of systems and process that gradually develop knowledge and confidence across all involved must be the aim, and this approach will ensure patient safety. It is clear that many of the mechanisms and process required to make the NHS patient-centred and to deliver the capacity and ability for self-care/management are in place. What is required is the courage and conviction through innovation and change management to deliver the processes across health and social care.

References

1. Department of Health (2009). *Operational Framework 2009/2010.* http://www. dh.gov.uk/prod_consum_dh/groups/dh_digitalassets/@dh/@en/documents/ digitalasset/dh_091446.pdf (accessed on October 2009).
2. Department of Health (2000). *The NHS Plan.* http://www.dh.gov.uk/prod_consum_ dh/groups/dh_digitalassets/@dh/@en/documents/digitalasset/dh_4055783.pdf (accessed on October 2009).
3. Wanless D (2002). *Securing Our Future Health: Taking a Long Term View. Final Report.* Department of Health. http://www.hm-treasury.gov.uk/consult_wanless_index.htm (accessed on October 2009).
4. Department of Health (2004). *Choosing Health: Making Healthy Choices Easier.* http://www.dh.gov.uk/prod_consum_dh/groups/dh_digitalassets/@dh/@en/ documents/digitalasset/dh_4105713.pdf (accessed on October 2009).
5. Department of Health (2009). *NHS Constitution.* http://www.dh.gov.uk/prod_ consum_dh/groups/dh_digitalassets/documents/digitalasset/dh_093442.pdf (accessed on October 2009).
6. Department of Health (2005). *Self Care – A Real Choice, Self Care Support – A Practical Option.* http://www.dh.gov.uk/prod_consum_dh/groups/dh_digitalassets/@dh/@en/ documents/digitalasset/dh_4101702.pdf (accessed on October 2009).
7. Department of Health (2001). *The Expert Patient.* http://www.dh.gov.uk/prod_ consum_dh/groups/dh_digitalassets/@dh/@en/documents/digitalasset/dh_ 4018578.pdf (accessed on October 2009).
8. Dorset and Somerset Strategic Health Authority (2006). *Promoting Optimal Self Care Consultation Techniques that Improve Quality of Life for Patients and Clinicians.* http:// www.swirl.nhs.uk/resource/164/ (accessed on October 2009).
9. Department of Health (2006). *Supporting People with Long Term Conditions: An NHS and Social Care Model to Support Local Innovation.* http://www.dh.gov.uk/prod_ consum_dh/groups/dh_digitalassets/@dh/@en/documents/digitalasset/dh_ 4122574.pdf (accessed on October 2009).
10. Department of Health and Skills for Care and Skills For Health (2008). *Common Core Principles to Support Self Care.* http://www.dh.gov.uk/prod_consum_dh/groups/ dh_digitalassets/@dh/@en/documents/digitalasset/dh_084506.pdf (accessed on October 2009).
11. Department of Health (2006). *Our Health, Our Care, Our Say.* http://www. dh.gov.uk/prod_consum_dh/groups/dh_digitalassets/@dh/@en/documents/ digitalasset/dh_4127459.pdf (accessed on October 2009).
12. Department of Health (2007). *Putting People First: A Shared Vision and Commitment to Transformation of Adult Social Care.* HMO Office http://www.dh.gov.uk/prod-con- sum_dh/groups/dh_digitalassets/@dh/@en/documents/digitalasset/dh_081119. pdf (accessed on October 2009).
13. National Institute for Health and Clinical Excellence (2005). *A Rapid Review of the Current State of Knowledge Regarding Lay-Led Self-Management of Chronic Illness: Evidence Review.* http://www.nice.org.uk/niceMedia/pdf/lay_led_rapid_review_ v10-FINAL.pdf (accessed on October 2009).
14. Institute for Healthcare Improvement (2005). *Chronic Conditions: Self Management: Changes for Improvement.* http://www.ihi.org/IHI/Topics/ChronicConditions/ AllConditions/Changes/ (accessed on October 2009).
15. Corben S and Rosen R (2005). *Self-Management for Long-Term Conditions: Patient's Perspectives on the Way Ahead.* King's Fund. http://www.kingsfund.org.uk/research/ publications/selfmanagement.html (accessed on October 2009).

16. Michie S, Miles J and Weinman J (2003). Patient centredness in chronic conditions: what does and does not matter? *Patient Education and Counselling*, 51, 197–206.
17. National Primary Care Research and Development Centre. *The WISE Approach to Self-Management University of Manchester 2007*. http://www.library.nhs.uk/PPI/ViewResource.aspx?resID=294441 (accessed on October 2009).
18. Central Cheshire Primary Care Trust (2006). *Working in Partnership Programme: Self Care for Primary Health Care Professionals Project*. http://www.wipp.nhs.uk/search.php?p=8&q=jusc
19. Primary Care Contracting, NHS (2007). *Primary Care Service Framework: Support for Self Care in Primary Care*. http://www.pcc.nhs.uk/uploads/medical/pcsf/primary_care_service_framework__self_care_v7_final.pdf (accessed on October 2009).
20. Dixon A (Ed.) (2007). *Engaging Patients in Their Health: How the NHS Needs to Change*. King's Fund. http://www.kingsfund.org.uk/research/publications/engaging_patients_in.html (accessed on October 2009).
21. Barlow JH, Wright C and Sheasby J (2002). Self management approaches for people with chronic conditions: a review. *Patient Education and Counselling*, 48, 177–187.
22. Sopel DR, Lorig KR and Hobbs M (2002). Chronic Disease Self-Management Programme: from development to dissemination. *The Permanente Journal*, 6(2), 15–22.
23. Wright CC, Barlow JH and Turner AP (2003). Self management training for people with chronic disease: an exploratory study. *British Journal of Health Psychology*, 8: 465–476 (ISSN 1359-107X).
24. Department of Health (2006). *Our Health, Our Care, Our Say: A New Direction for Community Services one year on*. http://www.dh.gov.uk/prod_consum_dh/groups/dh_digitalassets/@dh/@en/documents/digitalasset/dh_074522.pdf (accessed on October 2009).
25. Department of Health, Office of Public Management, GfK NOP and The University of York (August 2008). *Evaluation of Information on Prescriptions. Final Report*. http://www.dh.gov.uk/prod_consum_dh/groups/dh_digitalassets/@dh/@en/documents/digitalasset/dh_086888.pdf (accessed on October 2009).
26. Department of Health (2005). *Public Attitudes to Self-Care: Baseline Survey*. http://www.dh.gov.uk/prod_consum_dh/groups/dh_digitalassets/@dh/@en/documents/digitalasset/dh_4111263.pdf (accessed on October 2009).
27. Department of Health (2005). *Support for Self Care: A Practical Option Diagnostic, Monitoring and Assistive Tools, Devices, Technologies and Equipment to Support Self Care: Summary of a Review Report*. http://www.dh.gov.uk/prod_consum_dh/groups/dh_digitalassets/@dh/@en/documents/digitalasset/dh_4134014.pdf (accessed on October 2009).
28. Dixon A (2008). *Motivation and Confidence: What Does It Take to Change Behaviour?* King's Fund. http://www.kingsfund.org.uk/applications/site_search/?term=Motivation+and+Confidence%3A+What+Does+It+Take+to+Change+Behaviour%3F&searchreferer_id=2&submit.x=16&submit.y=10 (accessed on October 2009).
29. Boyce T, Robertson R and Dixon A (2008). *Commissioning and Behaviour Change: Kicking the Habits. Final Report*. King's Fund. http://www.kingsfund.org.uk/applications/site_search/?term=+Commissioning+and+Behaviour+Change%3A+Kicking+the+Habits.+Final+Report.&searchreferer_id=0&searchreferer_url=%2Fapplications%2Fsite_search%2Findex.rm&submit.x=10&submit.y=7 (accessed on October 2009).

Chapter 10
What Does This Mean for Patients?

Introduction

The main reason for implementation of a system of case management for long-term conditions is to improve the outcomes for patients and their carers. Although there is an understanding that there are potential benefits for the National Health Service (NHS) and social care services such as reduced use, or at least more effective use, of resources, in reality the key must be to reduce the negative impact long-term conditions have on people. The recent review by the NHS clearly describes the need for the NHS to focus its efforts on delivering the services that patients and their carers want, where they want them and in the ways they describe [1]. This is the era of modernisation, of care closer to home, of patient-centred care, of personalised budgets and of expectations of high quality in all services. Patients will no longer accept the excuse that because some care is delivered by health organisations and the rest by other agencies, it is difficult to ensure or enable continuity. The expectation is that care will be seamless, that it will be delivered to meet their needs and that it will be delivered when and where they want it; this is a high expectation indeed. This expectation means that services need to be commissioned and delivered based on the needs of patients in ways that reflect the views and preferences of patients. Access must be easy for patients and services must be available at times that are appropriate to patients, and not that suits the organisation of the service providers.

The health needs of the population of the future will continue to change; many of the diseases people develop cannot be cured but most can be managed. Developments in healthcare technology and treatments are increasing the number of disease that we can manage. The unhealthy choices we make as a population and the opportunities to improve health behaviours that have been missed over the recent past will continue to impact on needs unless robust action is taken quickly. The need for services that focus on personal needs to assist in reducing health inequalities is essential. Despite all of this, the need to ensure that all services we provide, be they preventative or care delivery, have added value and meet expectations is the current challenge for the NHS, both providers and commissioners.

Government expectations

The publication each year of an operating framework [2] that highlights for each year the key targets the NHS is expected to deliver in that year provides for commissioners guidance on what they need to commission in each financial or operating year. This year's operating framework in no different – this year the key targets for the NHS relate to the ability of the NHS to deliver patient-centred care and ensuring that choice is facilitated. In this chapter, patient experience and quality of services in both general and specific terms will be reviewed. The review of specific results of services for long-term conditions will probably assist in a broader understanding of the experience of being a patient in the NHS today, particularly as a person with complex health needs.

What do patients want from care?

The NHS is currently developing processes and policies that require increased performance information on services. This performance data and information must also be gathered based on the views of patients and staff regarding the outcomes of their care [3]. The patient-reported outcomes being debated and designed currently focus on outcomes in certain surgical procedures, but the expectation is that these will continue to be developed to cover a much boarder range of services and interventions. What is important to patients is the key to this debate and to the measurement of the effectiveness of services. Services already measure a number of metrics in relation to quality, but the majority of these measures are designed by professionals and are focused on the areas professionals believe are important. Although there may be some congruence between certain measures designed by professionals in for instance healthcare-acquired infection, it is highly likely that the views patients hold on good outcomes for them are personal to them and that they might be different from those of professionals.

   What is important to patients? Currently, we might not be 100% clear but we can postulate based on the feedback received during the recently held consultations regarding the future of the NHS and its modernisation. These consultations highlighted the importance placed by patients on wanting to be treated with respect. Although they are very concerned about cleanliness in hospitals and healthcare-acquired infections, they are also focused on how they are treated by the professionals. The important concepts of communication, respect, privacy and dignity are highly important, and also the ideas that they will be allowed to be involved and influence decisions on their care, which will be supported by appropriate information that would assist them and their carers in making decisions.

   The NHS Constitution [4] outlines for patients and the NHS the expectations on both sides. It is for the first time that a document describes what can be expected by patients (it could almost be described as a patients' bill of rights in relation to the NHS). This document also advises patients what the NHS has a right to expect in return – the concept of personal responsibility is very clearly outlined for all to see.

If all services are designed to meet the needs of a group of patients, then each service should have at its core a clear set of achievable goals, which it should be able to measure to evidence its level of effectiveness. These measures or goals must include the things that are important to patients and their carers, these could be described as patient reported outcomes. For case management the goals for professionals will be issues such as improved health outcomes, reduced emergency admissions, improved medication concordance and improved abilities for self-management by patients and carers. Some of these aims would be positively supported by patients without too much debate but the actual evidence of success in these aims may be viewed very differently by patients and carers and professionals. For the patient and carer success might be measured at a much lower level than a professional might wish.

Reported outcomes from management of long-term conditions

Reviews of case management by the King's Fund [5,6] have identified the key deliverable as improved functional status or prevention or slowing down of deterioration. For professionals this is an excellent outcome but for the patients and their carers the positive outcomes might be better described as a feeling of control over the disease or condition, or an improved understanding of the condition, and of course the improved continuity of care and provision of support to the patient and carers. Although these two sets of measures/outcomes could be seen as quite different, both have merit in that they are positive descriptions, and delivery against the patient expectations could provide a better base against which to measure the required professional outcomes. Patients and their carers are probably less interesting in saving the NHS resources through reduction of emergency admissions but would be extremely satisfied with any service that keeps them independent and improves their quality of life.

The ability of people to self-monitor and understand what the monitoring means and how they can influence their condition through making changes to the way they are living their lives would also be seen as empowering for both patients and their carers and would probably have a positive impact on health status. These processes are seen as allowing the patient and/or carers to understand how and when they need to access support for their condition and also what they may be able to do personally to improve their health [7].

The focus on improving health through education and empowerment, and of course providing high-quality care in a convenient way when people need it, is a positive step in health policy. This move from an illness service to a wellness service is a major cultural move for the NHS. But it is clear that people must understand the processes for both health and well-being, and how they can use them to the best advantage to make these positive moves effective. The message therefore must be one of identifying the way in which all services (preventative, rehabilitative and care) provide added value and make a real difference to patients' lives.

Modernisation to enable outcomes for users of services

As the design of services must be focused on the aspirations of patients, the current policies need to focus on how we ensure that we are engaging with patients and the public in determining the structure of local services, both health and social care. It is well known that making changes to the delivery of services that patients and carers understand, use and trust is unsettling for the service users, and there is a need for commissioners and providers to communicate effectively with patients and carers during any process that leads to service changes. Any change to service provision must be seen to add value to the patients' experience and must have been subject to robust debate and consultation processes. There is an expectation in the modern NHS that commissioners will evidence their ability to be 'world class' through this process [8] and recently all NHS commissioning organisations (primary care trusts [PCTs]) have completed their baseline assessment against the world class commissioning competencies.

'Creating a patient-led NHS' [9] published in 2005 identified for the NHS the concept of an NHS that responds to the needs of patients. The document outlines how the NHS would look if it was truly patient led. The concepts of information to enable choice are enshrined in the description, as is the requirement for robust safeguards for patients and delivery of high standards of care. The concept of the NHS organisation that can recognise needs of local people and design services to deliver for these needs in an innovative and different way is seen as absolutely essential. The concepts of patients in control of their care and the NHS delivering services that provide added value or positive impacts are also outlined as essential requirements of the NHS. The need for services to be provided with a culture based on concepts of dignity and respect is also highlighted as key requirements for both the commissioning and provision of care in the NHS. 'Our Health, Our Care, Our Say' [10] was developed following a wide consultation exercise with the public and describes the views and expectations of the public with regard to the design and delivery of health and social care services. Its seven key deliverables remain the foundation on which social care commissioning and care delivery are measured by regulators.

Do patients really see improvement?

In the same vein, the report on the next steps in the implementation of the National Service Framework for Older People [11] describes the progress made in improving services for older people including improvements in discharge planning and tackling discrimination, which has improved access to services. But the report also highlights the concerns that are still expressed by patients in relation to dignity in care.

Despite some real progress in services, the experiences reported by older people still highlight some unacceptable levels of care. The key areas of work identified in the report are as follows:

- Improvements in nutrition and the physical environment;
- Further development of skills, competence and leadership in the workforce;
- Assuring quality;
- Ensuring dignity at the end of life;
- Equalities and human rights;
- Championing change.

Help the Aged has produced a research report on dignity in care for older people [12]. The research was carried out to identify some of the possible indicators for dignity in care that could be utilised by service to measure delivery and success. The research has highlighted a set of draft indicators across the nine domains in dignity of care. The indicators identified as important are as follows:

- autonomy
- communication
- end-of-life care
- eating and nutrition
- pain
- personal hygiene
- personalised care
- privacy
- social inclusion

The domains outlined in relation to dignity of care are clearly useful in measuring what care feels like for the patient or service user. The ability of service provider to identify the level of autonomy a patient and/or their carer requires is highly important. It is clear that the providers of service must develop the skills needed to enable people who wish to be involved in the decision on their care to be so. The ability of staff to ascertain whether people wish to be involved in their care requires that they develop skills to identify what people wish to do for themselves and constantly review the understanding and arrangements. Involving people in their care when they wish to be involved or at the very least ensuring that their wishes and needs are taken into account when decision and plans are made must be an essential requirement for services as it is without doubt the principle on which consent is based. The ability of staff to enable people to take, when appropriate, responsibility for their own care, thereby promoting independence and choice, is essential. The ability of staff to promote independence allows patients to engage in social activities and make choices in relation to activities and relationships that can assist and further enable independence.

Help the Aged has produced for providers of service some excellent indicators and questions for users of services to enable measurement against these indicators. These have been developed as a tool that regulators and care providers could use to allow robust and effective measurement of the quality and effectiveness of care delivery specifically in relation to the issue of dignity in care provision. The indicators and measures have been designed with specific measure for specific care areas so this makes them valid and effective.

The ability to measure the user's experience of health or social care must be central to the delivery of high-quality care and of course the ability of service to maintain service quality. In the recent past, the Healthcare Commission (HCC) and Commission for Social Care Inspection (CSCI) now merged into the Care Quality Commission (CQC) have been accessing routinely the experience of users. Their reports highlight regularly that lack of dignity, lack of privacy and respect for confidentiality are major issues for patients. The level of frailty and disability of some patients can mean that those patients are highly vulnerable and may be less able to press for their rights. The Department of Health has been describing the need to promote the delivery of dignity in care for some years [13]. The research produced by Help the Aged continues this process through utilisation of the dignity domains developed by Levenson in 2007 [14] and through reviews of a number of studies carried out into people's accounts of dignity in the care they received. The research included the indicators identified in other documents and reports from organisations such as CSCI, Department of Health Essence of Care Framework [15], Help the Aged and the National Centre for Social Research. The researchers have outlined the challenges for dignity in care as:

- Over emphasis on targets and budgets that can militate against dignified care;
- The sacrifice of compassionate nursing care in the development of technical skills;
- Ageism in society and amongst healthcare staff.

The authors challenge the NHS and other service providers to take the issue of dignity and respect and make it a key agenda item for services, encouraging staff and all involved to make the issue an essential element of service provision.

Understanding the patient experience, how we find out?

How the NHS measures patient experience in an effective way is important. There have for some years been concerns across the NHS and its regulators regarding the ability and commitment of the NHS organisations to act appropriately and efficiently when the views of patients and carers are presented. The regulators of the NHS clearly define the need for organisations to evidence via the 'Standards for Better Health' declarations how they facilitate and enable patients' and carers' views and act on complaints and comments [16].

The HCC has since its inception had a key aim of involvement of the public and patients in their processes to assess the quality of health care for local areas. It has engaged with patients and the public to identify what matters to them and made sure that these influence how the annual health check of NHS organisations and service reviews are completed. The CQC and its predecessor the HCC have as a key aim to assess the quality of health care, which they then feed into these assessments and obtain the final ratings to enable a local focus and view. The information gathered is also used to evaluate the effectiveness of local health organisations in engaging their local population in decision making, prioritisation and service improvement processes. The organisations that utilise patients' views are seen as far more effective and score much better within the annual health check process.

The CQC access the views of patients and the public through a broad variety of ways [17]:

- The CQC helpline;
- The national programme of surveys of NHS patients;
- Workshops with the voluntary organisations that represent patient views;
- Working with patients and members of the public recruited to discuss specific issues;
- Invitations to local scrutiny committees and lay members of the boards of NHS foundation trusts and local involvement networks (LINks);
- Feedback from the SpeakOut network of community groups who are seldom listened to;
- Focus groups and online discussions with consultative panel of patients and members of the public.

The use of these processes allows the widest and most diverse levels of involvement and engagement and also encourages and enables the involvement of groups who might be seen as 'hard to reach' or who see themselves as unable to comment or become involved for a variety of reasons.

For the NHS to effectively meet the needs of patients it needs to recognise that patients are now much more demanding; they have higher levels of expectations than ever before. They want services that are convenient and accessible, delivered in way that is personalised to their needs. They require choice and influence on the care they receive – greater involvement in their care has been shown to improve the patients' experience and improve health outcomes [8]. One size definitely does not fit all. The latest guidance regarding the development of 'world class' commissioning competencies and abilities [18] focuses on a number of areas: the ability of commissioners to engage local people to identify the health needs, prioritise the needs and interventions and influence commissioning and procurement.

One of the many surveys completed by the NHS into services is the GP Patient Survey [19]; this survey was first completed in 2006/2007 and was used to assess the practice achievement of national standards set out in two Direct Enhanced Service agreements as part of the General Medical Services Contract.

The survey has provided to PCT commissioners information on levels of satisfaction with opening hours, and the 2007/2008 survey supported the development of extended opening hours in primary care. These surveys are delivered independently through Ipsos MORI and the questions used have been developed in partnership with primary care academics. The survey for 2008/2009 has been extended to include a broader question base, including environment, access to appointments, waiting time in surgery, seeing a preferred doctor and overall satisfaction with the care received. Further questions regarding management of long-term conditions and out of hours care will also be included in the survey. The survey will provide the evidence for achievement of the Quality and Outcomes Framework patient experience indicators for 2009/2010.

Public Service Agreement targets

The CQC has as part of the assessment process for the annual health check developed a range of metrics (new and existing targets also described as 'the vital signs'), which it uses to assess the quality of care and patient experience delivered by healthcare providers. These metrics are designed in disease-related groups (cancer, diabetes, urgent care, public health); each set of metrics includes a set of patient experience measures [20]. In October 2007, the PSA Delivery Agreement 19 was published [21] by the government. The aim for this agreement was to evidence the ongoing commitment to ensuring high quality, safe and accessible care that responds to the individual needs of patient is delivered across health and social care. The requirements of the Public Service Agreement (PSA) were focused on enabling the development and delivery of services with patients at the centre of planning. The progress against the PSA is monitored through eight key indicators.

Indicator 1, the self-reported experience of patients and users, identifies the need for robust information regarding experience of care to assist commissioners and providers to improve service provision. This is also thought to strengthen the ability of patients and users to influence the shape of service delivery. Evidence shows that a number of factors influence individuals' perception of their experience of care. These factors include accessibility, timeliness, quality, safety, effectiveness, dignity and respect. The policy aim for the NHS and social care is therefore to improve the overall experience for users, improving in those areas that are not meeting the required standards and consolidating on those areas where users do not raise concerns. The 'NHS Choices: Your Thoughts' website enables patients to comment on inpatient experiences.

Other assessments of user/patient experiences

In August 2007, the Health Foundation published 'Patient and public experiences' in the NHS [22], which focuses on quality and patient and public experience. The document reviews the policy documents published by the Department of Health since 2003 and tracks the reforms and commitments that relate to the delivery of a patient-centred NHS. The document also reflects on the significant increase in patient and public surveys that have been completed to inform the development of policy and services. The reviewed surveys report that in general terms the public values the service provided by the NHS, with three-quarters of patients rating the care received as excellent or good.

The use of consultation to influence health policy is evident through the results of the national choice consultation completed in 2003, which identified that 76% of respondents thought the most important aspect of NHS care was involving patients in decisions about treatment. A number of other surveys reviewed in this report describe the most important attributes for the NHS as being:

- Affordable treatment and care, free at the point of care;
- Safety and quality;
- Health protection and disease prevention;
- Accessible local services and national centres of excellence;
- Universal coverage; geographical and social equity;
- Responsiveness, flexibility and choice;
- Participation in service development;
- Transparency, accountability and opportunity to influence policy decisions.

The Picker Institute published in 2007 the results of a survey that provided information on how patients scored 82 different aspects of care. The most important aspects for patient were those relating to cleanliness (doctors and nurses washing their hands and rooms appearing clean), staff who understand the patients' condition and who can answer questions appropriately and communication skills (the ability of staff to explain options for care including risks and benefits) [23]. None of these should be a surprise to professionals as they relate very clearly to the need of patients to be in control of their destiny and feel confident of the care they are receiving. The expectations of patients accessing primary care services are similar: professionals explaining clearly, giving time to give information and ensuring confidentiality.

The areas that have been identified as important to the public and patients outline for the NHS the need to move away from the traditional model of viewing the patient as passive within the health partnership, or as holding the assumption that the professional knows best. This is not how patients and public now expect to be treated; patients and carers expect to be involved in decisions and have an expectation that their views and preferences will be taken into account when deciding care. There is growing evidence that involving patients and enabling them to self-manage and self-care leads to more effective and appropriate use of services and resources.

In 2006 the HCC undertook a survey of people with diabetes in which they asked the patients their level of involvement in decision, the education provided, the information they received at diagnosis and the explanations provided regarding medication; positive responses regarding these processes are known to evidence good-quality care and to lead to improvements in patient outcomes. The issue of safety and protection against unnecessary risks and harm is also important to patients and the public. The issues in the NHS with healthcare-acquired infection, medication issues owing to poly-pharmacy and learning from incidents and complaints are all identified as important areas of concern for patients and the public.

Patient-centred health care is the policy requirement, and is an ideal to which all would agree the NHS and social care must aim. Social care, which has a longer history of aiming to deliver personalised care and user involvement, is still striving to achieve. The Commission for Social Care Inspection in 2006 [23] outlined for social care the requirements of user involvement and user centeredness. The report defines for care providers the most effective ways in which to empower people, and of course how to ensure that we can provide care in a way that is valued. They also outline the requirements for commissioners to build a provider market, through working to develop providers that are user led and focused. This report also suggests that user involvement must be supported to enable a challenge the status quo, assist in setting the agenda and contribute to how decisions are made.

The commission argues that the only way to become user focused is to regard the user as 'king', understanding what the user wants and needs and delivering it. The needs and expectations of service users and carers should drive changes and developments in services. As users take control of how their care is delivered and arranged, their relationship with care providers (NHS or social care) will change, and therefore the role of professionals should become one of a facilitator of care. One of the key roles of case management is to orchestrate and facilitate care supporting the patient to ensure that care is delivered in an appropriate way and at the level the patient expects; this is all about ensuring that the patient/user experience is positive.

It is argued that the case for focusing on the patient experience and deciding how to improve the experiences is a moral and human imperative [24]. This will ensure that we can protect people who are vulnerable and weak, and promote quality and humanity in care. It is argued that the aim to improve experience is justified on both clinical and value for money grounds. Good communication with patients improves concordance, enables understanding, enhances self-care, increases confidence and provides a feeling of well-being for patients. The information regarding the experience of patients within services and organisations will in the longer term impact on the choices patients make regarding where and how to access care. The requirement for quality reports from all providers [1] and the impact of these reports on the annual health check and other reports produced by regulators such as the newly formed Care Quality Commission should not be underestimated. The Care Quality Commission has clearly described that quality reports will be treated as having the same level of importance as the yearly financial reports expected from organisations.

Patient-centred care

Patient-centred as defined in the King's Funds report [24] implies the development of a common vision for care, a vision that ensures that patients' views are central to planning of their care. The concept of patient-centred care is subject to enormous debate amongst practitioners. Some service areas, such as primary care, can conceptualise the model more easily than others. As primary care considers the social and psychological perspectives in care, it focuses on the meaning of illness for individuals and the need to negotiate shared responsibility for decision making and action, and it recognises the influence of personal qualities on patients and how they react. In cancer services and the management of long-term condition, patient-centred care focuses on management models that identify what patients think, believe and expect in their care.

Allowing patients to tell their tale

Point of care defines the patient experiences not as the remit of professionals but as a product of the whole system [25]. The experience relates to whole journey, every interaction and contact across the course of care, and this will include clinical and non clinical staff, all support services and even the senior managers. Everyone contributes to the quality of the patients' experience. It is essential that we listen to the patient; the only way we can understand how it feels is to accept that the patient is the only one with a true view on what it feels like.

Listening to the stories from patients can bring the reality of care alive; for many years patients have attempted to communicate their views in a broad range of ways (paintings, memoirs, films, fiction). Patients have used the Internet and the media to tell their tales. These can be harrowing, intense and uncomfortable to hear.

The key issue in the reports of patient experience is the problem of variability in quality and experience. Often the experience will be excellent at one time and poor at another, depending on the staff available at the time. The importance of the patient being seen as person cannot be underestimated; patients' stories have a unique ability to provide insight into the relationship between the care process and what it feels like for the patient. In 2007, patient survey by the HCC reported that 92% of patients rated their care as excellent, very good or good, with a steadily increasing number of patients who rate their care as excellent.

Outcomes of care and patient experience

As outlined earlier, the expectations the public have of health care are changing, and this is particularly true of patients in their 60s [26]. The aspirations of the 'baby boomers' (those born between 1945 and 1954) are viewed as very different to those of previous generations. The key difference being that this generation has an expectation of greater choice, higher quality, improved involvement and equality of access (rooting out discrimination). These older people are no longer seen as passive users of services, they must be viewed as members of the population who wish to make a continued contribution. Communities that have a culture of valuing their older people with an expectation that these people have a positive contribution to their communities are seen as enabling positive life experiences for their older people. 'Living well in later life' [27] outlines that during their review 80% of older people who were asked reported that they do not think that they have influenced service planning or delivery, this despite the requirement with the National Service Framework for Older People to involve older people in these processes. The review reported that while older people value the services they receive and feel that they are being treated with dignity and respect, there are still reports of some areas where dignity, respect and sensitivity are lacking in service provisions. More worryingly, the report identifies some high numbers (in one area 27% and in another area 59%) of people who felt reluctant to complain or were not confident that the complaint would be listened to. The report identified a number of areas in which older people still have major concerns: provision of information, communication skills, the ability or willingness of staff to take time to answer questions and the promotion of active involvement by patients in care planning. These areas remain problematic despite evidence that improvements in these areas would make a major difference to both care outcomes and patient experience.

The Wanless Review [28] clearly defines that there is a important difference between capturing information on processes and measurement of outcomes as these are described as recording the first-hand experience of users. The measurement of performance in services is through outcomes achieved, but the measurement of outcomes is complex as outcomes for users are influenced by decisions and preferences through which service users make choices regarding care. The Relative Needs Survey reviewed by Wanless discusses the outcomes reported by people using services and also if they did not use the service. The aim was to measure what is described as outcome gain – the difference between before and after services.

Interestingly, the working paper from the King's Fund [29], which reports the views of older people, outlines the personal priorities for improved care. It does not focus on care services per se but outlines the importance of transport, leisure and education opportunities as essential underpinnings of care, alongside advocacy to enable patients to access entitlements. The people involved in the process for this report while agreeing that care provision is important describe that very often the problems in meeting social needs (availability of transport, advocacy, etc.) actually outweighed their care needs.

All local councils are expected to ensure that users complete satisfaction surveys; in the main, these ask questions of patients regarding the level of satisfaction with service provision (service use, quality number of hours of contact). The national results report that 57% of users are very or extremely satisfied. Users who reported increased independence levels are likely to report significant levels of gain in relation to outcomes.

Experience in case management

Patient and carers in receipt of case management/services to manage long-term conditions are often asked to state their views on the services they receive. All areas that have piloted or implemented case management models of care have completed some form of effectiveness review/evaluation. Most of these have included patient and carer views alongside professional and stakeholder views.

Views from patients and carers in relation to case management models have been positive. The report 'Improving care for older people with long-term conditions' [29], which reviewed the frameworks for managing long-term conditions in the United Kingdom and internationally, highlights that evaluations have provided evidence that patients report an increased feeling of control, increased information about their condition and control and improved experience of care. The improvements in experience of care included care quality, consistency, accessibility, reduction in complaints and improved quality of life. All of which are highly positive for the patient and carers. Specific evaluations completed describe patients and carers feeling for the first time being finally in control or of having a professional who was listening to problems and issues and taking positive action [30].

All care management programmes have defined clearly principles that include the aim of 'providing individualised, whole person approach to care' or some very similar aim, which are highly relevant in light of recent policy drivers. It is very clear from the review of intensive care management in Peterborough [31] that the experience of patients and carers of case management models is positive. The patient and carers provided very positive feedback in relation to an improved feeling of support and continuity of management, better understanding of condition and confidence that issues would be managed effectively and a feeling of 'someone is interested in them'. As part of the evaluation into the service for patients receiving case management in Haringey [32] criteria being reviewed are improved health behaviours, improved self-care, more appropriate use of services and satisfaction with care received.

In the Evercare review [33], two-thirds of patients and carers reported improvements in quality of care when in receipt of case management. The improvements outlined by patients included improved coping abilities and quality of life. All patient and carers reported high level of satisfaction with the personalised care planning process, which enabled all areas of care need to be understood and appropriately planned and supported. Ninety-five per cent of patients and carers reported being involved in the decision relating to care and 97% reported that they felt they had enough time to discuss health or medical problems and that the nurse provided information and explanations of reasons for treatment in an understandable way. Patients also reported that the provision of case management reduced anxiety regarding their condition and their ability to cope with long-term problems through enabling patients and carers to recognise when condition is changing and requires action. Patients and carers reported very positive perceptions of care provided (96%) in the review of

Evercare and over 98% reported that they had been treated with respect and dignity. The evaluation also highlighted similar levels (98%) of confidence and trust in the nurses providing care and advice. With 90% of patients and carers feeling that the nurses communicated well and worked well with both patients and carers to plan care. Ninety-five per cent of patients reported increased ability to understand, manage and cope with their disease and more than 50% felt their quality of life had improved, with just under a quarter (24%) reporting significant improvement in quality of life.

The Department of Health has published a number of key documents that outline the expectations for patient outcomes for case management. Raising the profile of long-term conditions care [34] describes some high level outcomes:

- Improved quality of life, health and well-being and enablement to be independent;
- Supported and enabled to self-care and actively involved in decisions;
- Choice and control over care and service, which are built around individual including carer needs;
- Integrated, flexible, proactive and responsive care;
- High-quality, efficient and sustainable care.

Other key outcomes for patients in receipt of case management are reported as promotion and maintenance of independence, the ability to maintain links with communities and to be able to be active in the community. This feeling of independence and continued involvement in social activities does appear to have a huge impact on patients and carers.

All evaluations of case management services, alongside many other services, outline the impact of attitudes of staff and the need for excellent communication skills to ensure the delivery of high-quality care and meeting patients' expectations. Key issues for patients and carers relate to the ability of staff to treat them with respect and courtesy, the issue of sensitivity in communication is also highly important to patients and carers. Some of the evaluations of case management models have reported high levels of effectiveness and improved outcomes for patients and carers where integration of health and social care has been in place whether virtual or full. The models of care used in social care are often described as highly person centred as every person is assessed as an individual and a care plan developed, which the service user or carer usually 'signs up' or agrees to; the arrangements for delivery of care in this area are obviously slightly different owing to the 'means testing' for access to delivery as against a free at the point of care process used within the NHS. Despite these differences, the NHS has much to learn from social care in relation to involvement in care decisions and from the process social care managers use to assess effectiveness of care packages, which includes service users and carers at every stage of the review and has an expectation that the comments and views received will underpin all future plans for service delivery. The outcome of the support provided to enable carers, and other members of the patients support network, to cope with the pressures and requirements placed upon them is the key to effectiveness of the service. The ability of carers and support networks to manage caring responsibilities in a positive way, which allows them to maintain social contacts and keeps them well, is essential as these carers provide essential support for patient independence, as well as the care that would be required via health and social care providers if they were not available.

Partnerships with patients: impact on experience

Partnerships with patients and carers are without doubt a key process in delivering effective care for patients with long-term conditions; through these partnerships the services could develop specific measures for individuals, which enable ownership of the care plan and may increase levels of concordance. The report from the International Alliance of Patient Organisations [35] has reviewed the research available into the views of and expectations of patients in relation to patient-centred care. Although this review identified a number of definitions for patient-centred care and reported these as dependent on the culture and context in which patients were living, all descriptions verbalise the need for information and partnership to enable and understand 'what the patient needs and wants'.

The requirement of partnership is essential in enabling and ensuring control for patients and service users, and successful delivery in the pilots of individual health budgets will be heavily dependent on partnership with service users as without this safety and effectiveness of services may be difficult to maintain. The ability of staff to communicate effectively with patients and carers, providing information that is understandable and clear to support agreements of plans and outcomes will support this process, and while the issues relating to information provision and sharing with patients have been reviewed elsewhere, it remains important to note here the importance of this process across the area of long-term conditions care. The delivery of services in a personalised way, while maintaining the standards (following appropriate protocols), requires staff who are highly skilled and hold high levels of professional judgement to ensure that effective information is provided to enable appropriate decisions to be made with patients.

Outcomes in the services that reach out to communities promoting healthy behaviours and personal responsibility particularly with disadvantaged groups will be a continuing challenge for the NHS and social care, as most of these services will require members of the population to change deeply engrained health behaviours such as smoking and alcohol intake, so outcomes for these may require some innovative thinking during development. Despite the possible challenges, much work has been done with children and young people to develop different expectations in families in relation to health that may provide some innovative measures to use. The ever increasing focus in government policy on prevention of ill-health through preventive services and promotion of self-care requires that all services have some focus on providing prevention with either the service users, the families, carers or staff; evidence of outcomes will be long-term but the delivery is essential to reduce the impact of ill-health on the population. The NHS of the future will need to change its focus from responding and reacting to proactively identifying health issues and provision of service and processes to mitigate health risks working always with local populations to define expectations and possible models of delivery.

The ever changing nature of disease and the development in information technology will effect the expectations on service delivery in the future. Many of the services of future will be delivered via mobile technology – monitoring and providing support for long-term conditions via telemedicine is well established in many areas. The patient outcomes for these services will be focused on the ability of the support to keep the patient well, the safety of the process and the confidence the service user has in the service provision.

The expected impact of increasing numbers of older people requiring health and social care means that we need to plan for services for the future. The ability to predict services required is dependent on an understanding of the outcomes the services will need to deliver. The perceived outcomes and benefits received by users from a service are influenced by the level of dependence. It remains clear though that there are some fundamental expectations on service provision. The expectation that service users will be safe and protected is one of these. The ability of a service to provide the wherewithal for a patient to enjoy a fulfilling life (social inclusion and involvement and self-esteem and well-being) is also essential. Another expectation is that any service has the ability to provide support for carers, enabling them to live a normal life free of undue stress. These expectation were developed as part of the consultation for 'Our health, our care, our say' [10] and remain relevant today.

Quality for patients

The view of the Department of Health is that for patients quality is what matters [1] and while this may seem an obvious statement, it is clear that a definition of what quality might mean to patients is fundamental to the debate. The department in consultation with patients has defined the areas of quality that are important to patients. The NHS review outlined what patients described as quality:

- Treatment that is effective;
- Keep patients as safe as possible;
- Help patients stay healthy (working in partnership to promote health);
- Empower patients (give people rights and control over care).

These quality issues are enshrined as requirements on which the NHS needs to deliver and on which the NHS will be performance managed in delivery.

Inspirational leadership is seen as the framework on which improvements in services will be delivered [36]. Clinical ownership of quality processes is crucial to delivery. The development of clinical leadership is one of the foundation stones on which improvements in services are dependent; the move towards an agenda with the patient at the centre and quality as a key expectation is seen as providing an opportunity to mobilise and empower clinicians as well as patients. This desire for quality improvement means that clinical leadership needs to be a key function in everything we do. Potential leaders must be identified and nurtured with appropriate support for skill development.

A wide variety of terms have been used to define quality including humanity, efficiency, effectiveness, equity, acceptability, appropriateness and accessibility. The Institute of Medicine in the United States developed the definition that is recognised internationally [24]; this definition has six criteria: patient-centred, safe, effective, timely, efficient and equitable. Currently, the term of choice in improvement literature in relation to quality is patient-centred.

Impact of the provision of information on patients' views and outcomes

The evaluation information on prescription pilots [37] outlined the intended and actual impact of this information process. The intended outcomes relate to improved patient experience, improved quality of life and better clinical outcomes. The evaluation describes that 95% of users made use of the information provided, and a large majority of users reported finding the information useful, although the figures were lower in disadvantaged areas. Seventy-three per cent of the users involved reported increased levels of confidence when dealing with professionals and 52% felt that the information they received helped to improve their care. Sixty-six per cent felt more in control of their condition, though surprisingly 59% of users reported that they would prefer to be told what to do rather than finding information to make decisions themselves. This evaluation does highlight though that during the pilot processes users in disadvantaged areas or marginalised groups found the information prescriptions less useful than users in other areas and groups.

Conclusions

Across the developing world, governments and organisation are asking similar questions, what does care need to look like, how do we deliver to meet the needs and what will services look like to ensure sustainability? Perhaps the question should be what service do people want and need? This chapter has attempted to focus on the later question particularly in relation to what people in receipt of care really describe as important to them whatever the setting or service. The recent review [1] of the NHS outlined the need to take on board the differing views and needs of people across local communities in designing and delivering services. The emphasis of health care is moving from treatment as defined in 1948 to improving health and promoting and extending 'wellness'; this process is making delivery more complex. The need to shape services around the requirements and needs of local populations will be a challenge and it is expected that this will mean that while access will be universal, provision may not be uniform, so services may be designed and delivered specifically to meet an area's needs. It is hoped that this flexibility will enable a focus for service development in areas where health equalities are at the highest.

Although it is clear that ensuring patient expectation and choice is highly important, there remains a need to ensure that these processes are provided within a safe environment. For example, choice to appropriate care must be enabled through information that the patient or carer can understand and use appropriately. Choice will enable the people to have control, but this must be enabled while respecting individual lifestyle choices and preferences and with the ability of the people to be as involved as they are comfortable with in decision making. Although not everyone will want to be involved every time a decision is made, the opportunity to do so is surely a fundamental human right. The attitude of staff is a major issue for service provision – almost all complaints within services have as a key area of concern the attitude of staff and communication skills. For quality and outcomes to improve, communication and staff attitudes must improve, and to do this organisations must engage staff at all levels and win the hearts and minds in the promotion of good care. All staff have a vested interest as potential users, or relatives of users of services, in the quality and outcomes of all services. All staff must be engaged in the development and implementation of service quality and patient outcomes processes because they will understand the 'real world' issues that affect service provision. This does not mean that the status quo in services should not be challenged, as for the modernisation of services to be effective a robust challenge must come from all. Personalisation of care does appear to be one of the most effective processes to enable the delivery of care in line with patient needs and expectations. The ability of the NHS to commission services in this way, and of all service providers to deliver in this way, remains a work in progress.

The ability to really measure what is important to patients, while at the same time measuring and reporting the measures required to evidence effective health impact, remains something of a challenge for services. The requirement to design and deliver services with patients at the centre must, therefore, push reporting of effectiveness and outcomes towards the views and expectations of patients themselves. The need to link the patient-reported measures to some form of effectiveness measures in line with NHS policy such as value for money or reduction of emergency service use will require some innovative thought, but is not impossible. We must though maintain some focus on patients' experience and outcomes as if the drive towards person-centred care is to be a reality, then we must be able to report what care really feels like for the individual and if we are not able or willing to do this, then perhaps person-centred care will never be a delivered in real terms.

References

1. Department of Health (2008). *High Quality Care for All: NHS Next Stage Review. Final Report*. http://www.dh.gov.uk/prod_consum_dh/groups/dh_digitalassets/@dh/@en/documents/digitalasset/dh_085828.pdf (accessed on October 2009).

2. Department of Health (2009). *Operating Framework for the NHS 2009/2010*. http://www.dh.gov.uk/prod_consum_dh/groups/dh_digitalassets/@dh/@en/documents/digitalasset/dh_091446.pdf (accessed on October 2009).

3. Department of Health (2009/2010). *Patient-Reported Outcomes*. http://www.dh.gov.uk/prod_consum_dh/groups/dh_digitalassets/@dh/@en/documents/digitalasset/dh_092625.pdf (accessed on October 2009).

4. Department of Health (2009). *NHS Constitution*. http://www.dh.gov.uk/prod_consum_dh/groups/dh_digitalassets/documents/digitalasset/dh_093442.pdf (accessed on October 2009).

5. Dixon J, Lewis R, Rosen R, Finlayson B and Gray D (2004). *Managing Chronic Disease: What We Can Learn from the US Experience*. King's Fund. http://www.kingsfund.org.uk/research/publications/managing_chronic.html (accessed on October 2009).

6. Warner J, Lewis R and Gillam S (2001). *US Managed Care and PCTs: Lessons from a Small Island to a Lost Continent*. King's Fund. http://www.kingsfund.org.uk/applications/site_search/?term=US+Managed+Care+and+PCTs%3A+Lessons+from+a+Small+Island+to+a+Lost+Continent&searchreferer_id=10204&submit.x=40&submit.y=6 (accessed on October 2009).

7. Department of Health (2008). *A High-Quality Workforce: NHS Next Stage Review*. http://www.dh.gov.uk/prod_consum_dh/groups/dh_digitalassets/@dh/@en/documents/digitalasset/dh_085841.pdf (accessed on October 2009).

8. Kendall L (2007). *What Needs to Change to Meet the Needs of Future Patients?* King's Fund http://www.kingsfund.org.uk/applications/site_search/?term=Needs+to+Change+to+Meet+the+Needs+of+Future+Patients&searchreferer_id=2&submit.x=10&submit.y=14

9. Department of Health (2005). *Creating a Patient-Led NHS: Delivering the NHS Improvement Plan*. http://www.dh.gov.uk/prod_consum_dh/groups/dh_digitalassets/@dh/@en/documents/digitalasset/dh_4106507.pdf (accessed on October 2009).

10. Department of Health (2006). *Our Health, Our Care, Our Say: A New Direction for Community Services*. http://www.dh.gov.uk/prod_consum_dh/groups/dh_digitalassets/@dh/@en/documents/digitalasset/dh_4127459.pdf (accessed on October 2009).

11. Department of Health (2006). *A New Ambition for Old Age: Next Steps in Implementing the National Service Framework for Older People*. http://www.dh.gov.uk/prod_consum_dh/groups/dh_digitalassets/@dh/@en/documents/digitalasset/dh_4133947.pdf (accessed on October 2009).

12. Magee H, Parsons S and Askham J (2008). *Measuring Dignity in Care for Older People. A Research Report for Help the Aged*. Picker Institute Europe. http://policy.helptheaged.org.uk/NR/rdonlyres/EFD769F8-930A-412E-B079-FD058EE6AA69/0/on_our_own_terms_021208.pdf (accessed on October 2009).

13. Department of Health (2006). *Dignity in Care Campaign*. http://www.dh.gov.uk/prod_consum_dh/groups/dh_digitalassets/@dh/@en/documents/digitalasset/dh_065426.pdf (accessed on October 2009).

14. Levenson R (2007). *The Challenge of Dignity in Care*.

15. Department of Health (2003). *Essence of Care*. http://www.dh.gov.uk/prod_consum_dh/groups/dh_digitalassets/@dh/@en/documents/digitalasset/dh_4127915.pdf

16. Healthcare Commission (July 2004). *Standards for Better Health*. http://www.dh.gov.uk/prod_consum_dh/groups/dh_digitalassets/@dh/@en/documents/digitalasset/dh_4132991.pdf (accessed on October 2009).

17. Department of Health & Care Quality Commission (2001). *Involving Patients and the Public*. http://www.dh.gov.uk/prod_consum_dh/groups/dh_digitalassets/@dh/@en/documents/digitalasset/dh_088803.pdf.   http://www.cqc.org.uk/_db/_documents/A4_Report_2009_01.pdf (accessed on October 2009).

18. Department of Health (2008). *Commissioning Assurance Handbook: World Class Commissioning 'Adding Life to Years and Years to Life'*. http://www.dh.gov.uk/prod_consum_dh/groups/dh_digitalassets/@dh/@en/documents/digitalasset/dh_085141.pdf (accessed on October 2009).

19. Department of Health (2008). *The GP Patient Survey Guidance for Strategic Health Authorities, Primary Care Trusts and GP Practice: The New Expanded GP Patient Survey 2008/09*. http://www.dh.gov.uk/prod_consum_dh/groups/dh_digitalassets/@dh/@en/documents/digitalasset/dh_092087.pdf (accessed on October 2009).

20. Healthcare Commission (2007). *The Better Metrics Project*. http://www.cqc.org.uk/_db/_documents/Better_Metrics_full_report.pdf (accessed on October 2009).

21. HM Government (2007). *Public Service Agreements Delivery Agreement 19: Ensure Better Care for All*. http://www.hm-treasury.gov.uk/pbr_csr07_psaindex.html (accessed on October 2009).

22. Leatherman S and Sutherland K (2007). *Patient and Public Experience in the NHS Quest for Quality and Improved Performance*. The Health Foundation. http://www.health.org.uk/publications/research_reports/patient_and_public.html (accessed on October 2009).

23. Commission for Social Care Inspection (2006). *Relentless Optimism Creative Commissioning for Personalised Care*. http://www.ofsted.gov.uk/Ofsted-home/Publications-and-research/Browse-all-by/Documents-by-type/Thematic-reports/Relentless-optimism-creative-commissioning-for-personalised-care (accessed on October 2009).

24. Goodrich J and Cornwell J (2008). *Seeing the Person in the Patient. The Point of Care Review Paper*. King's Fund. http://www.kingsfund.org.uk/research/publications/the_point_of_care.html (accessed on October 2009).

25. King's Fund (2005). *Social Care Needs and Outcomes: The Wanless Social Care Review*. http://www.kingsfund.org.uk/research/projects/wanless_social_care_review/ (accessed on October 2009).

26. Commission for Social Care Inspection, Audit Commission and Healthcare Commission (2006). *Living Well in Later Life: A Review of Progress Against the National Service Framework for Older People*. http://www.audit-commission.gov.uk/health/nationalstudies/socialcare/Pages/livingwellinlaterlife_copy.aspx#downloads (accessed on October 2009).

27. Wanless D (2006). *Securing Good Care for Older People Taking a Long Term View*. King's Find. http://www.kingsfund.org.uk/research/publications/securing_good.html (accessed on October 2009).

28. Levenson R, Jeyasingham M, and Joule N (2005). *Looking Forward to Care in Old Age. Expectations of the Next Generation*. King's Fund. http://www.kingsfund.org.uk/applications/site_search/?term=Looking+Forward+to+Care+in+Old+Age.+Expectations+of+the+Next+Generation&searchreferer_id=2&submit.x=33&submit.y=6 (accessed on October 2009).

29. University of Birmingham (HSMC) and NHS Institute for Innovation and Improvement (2006). *Improving Care for People with Long-Term Conditions: A Review of UK and International Frameworks*. http://www.improvingchroniccare.org/downloads/review_of_international_frameworks__chris_hamm.pdf (accessed on October 2009).

30. Bristol South and West, Bristol North and South Gloucestershire Primary Care Trusts (2004). *The Bristol & South Gloucestershire Evercare Programme Report.* http://www. networks.nhs.uk/39 (accessed on October 2009).
31. Greater Peterborough Primary Care Partnership and King's Find (2007). *Intensive Care Management.* http://www.kingsfund.org.uk/applications/site_search/?term= Greater+Peterborough&searchreferer_id=0&searchreferer_url=%2Fapplications% 2Fsite_search%2Findex.rm&submit.x=5&submit.y=11
32. Haringey PCT and King's Fund (2007). *TeamHealth: Long Term Condition Partnership Pilot between Haringey Teaching Primary Care Trust and Pfizer.* http://www.networks. nhs.uk/39 (accessed on October 2009).
33. UnitedHealth Europe (2005). *Assessment of the Evercare Programme in England 2003–2004.* http://www.dh.gov.uk/prod_consum_dh/groups/dh_digitalassets/@dh/@en/ documents/digitalasset/dh_4114224.pdf (accessed on October 2009).
34. Department of Health (2008). *Raising the Profile of Long Term Conditions Care: A Compendium of Information.* http://www.dh.gov.uk/prod_consum_dh/groups/dh_ digitalassets/documents/digitalasset/dh_082067.pdf (accessed on October 2009).
35. International Alliance of Patient Organisations (2007). *What is Patient Centred Healthcare? A Review of Definitions and Principles.* http://www.patientsorganizations. org/pchreview (accessed on October 2009).
36. Department of Health (2008). *Inspiring Leaders: Leadership for Quality Guidance for NHS Talent and Leadership Plans.* http://www.dh.gov.uk/prod_consum_dh/groups/dh_ digitalassets/documents/digitalasset/dh_093407.pdf (accessed on October 2009).
37. Department of Health Office of Public Management, GfK and University of York (2008). *Evaluation of Information on Prescription. Final Report.* http://www. informationprescription.info/finalreport.html (accessed on October 2009).

Index

Adult Social Service, 35, 167
advanced care planning, 139–40
advanced clinical nursing practice, 45,
        47–9, 85–91, 133
advanced practice
    definition, 157
    and leadership, 144, 157–8
    in long-term conditions, 159–60
Alaskan Medical Service, 22–3
Amsterdam HealthCare System, 27
Anthem Blue Cross and Blue Shield, 22, 26
Australian model of care, for chronic
        diseases, 28

'baby boomer generation', 107, 195
Barnsley PCT, 35

cancer care and end-of-life care, patient
        outcomes for, 123
    advanced care planning, 139–40
    case management
        competencies, 132–7
        and ICCP, 131–2
    competencies, need for, 137–8
    delivering choice programmes, 140
    Gold Standards Framework (GSF), for
        palliative care, 125
    ICCP, 125–7
    pilot programmes
        delivering, 129
        preparing for, 127–9
    preferred place of care, 140
    programme outcomes, 130–31
care delivery, 113
    and case management, 10–11
    in NHS, 11–13
care management, 36, 38, 105, 113, 197
    development, 12
    in social care, 32
Care Orchestration, 11, 26, 49–50
Care Quality Commission, 148, 194
CARMEN network, 107
Centre for Health Studies, 25

chronic care model, 10, 25, 29
    in United States, 20
chronic disease
    impact and cost, 6–7
    management, 9–10
Chronic Disease Management Program, 174
chronic long-term conditions,
        management of, 1
clinical leadership, 94, 154, 201
    and organisational leadership, 144
Cochrane Collaboration, 5
cognitive impairment and mental
        well-being, management of, 52–4,
        134–5
Commission for Social Care Inspection,
        190, 194
Community Care Act (1990), 18, 32
community matron, 28, 35, 44, 48, 62, 94,
        102, 129, 136–7, 141, 159
competence, 132–7
    of case management, 132–7
    definition, 43–4
    and deliverables, for patients/service
        users
        leading complex care co-ordination,
            66–74
    educational models, for competency
        development, 62–4
    levels, 150
    for managing long-term conditions, 43
        advanced clinical nursing practice,
            47–9
        aim, 61–2
        cognitive impairment and mental
            well-being, management of, 52–4
        competency framework, development
            of, 44–6
        complex long-term conditions,
            management of, 52, 53
        educational models to develop
            competencies, 62–4
        end-of-life care, 59–60
        expectations, delivery of, 46

competence (*Continued*)
    health promotion and ill health
        prevention, 58–9
    high-risk people, identification of,
        58–9
    interagency and partnership working,
        60–61
    leading complex care co-ordination,
        49–51
    professional practice and leadership,
        57–8
    self-care, self-management and
        enabling independence, 55–6
    need for, 137–8
    of practitioners, 39
competency framework, development of,
    44–6
complex care co-ordination, 49–51, 66–74,
    133–4
complex care management, patient
    outcomes on, 66
    competence and deliverables, 66–74
    high-risk patients identification, health
        promotion and ill health
        prevention, 74–7
    interagency and partnership working,
        77–82
complex long-term conditions,
    management of, 52, 53
Comprehensive Area Assessment (CAA),
    97
cost of care, for older people, 109–11
Croydon PCT, 37

Darzi Review, 10, 96, 142, 153
data, for case management, 38
'delivering choice programmes', 140
Department of Health (DH), 1, 2, 12, 20, 32,
    105, 125–6, 141, 142, 178, 190, 198
Dutch healthcare system, 22, 27

East Lincolnshire PCT, 36
end-of-life care, 59–60, 97–8, 124, 135–7
England
    models in use in, 30–31
    NHS in, 1
EPIC (Elderly Care Project in Cornwall)
    report, 36
evaluations, of case management models,
    38–40
Evercare programme, 11, 26, 155

evidence base, for lay-led
    self-management, 173–5
Expanded Chronic Care Model, 29
experience, in case management, 197–9
Expert Patient Programme (EPP), 13, 165,
    168–9, 170
    and self-management programmes, 169

facilitative leadership, 153
Foster Intelligence, 7
FSS/Relative Needs survey, 196

General Medical Services contract, 2,
    4, 191
Gold Standards Framework (GSF), for
    palliative care, 125
'good health', definition of, 123
government expectations, 186
GP Patient Survey, 191
Greater Peterborough Primary Care Trust
    Partnership, 37, 197
Green Ribbon Health, 22, 30
Group Health Cooperative, 22, 25
Guided Care, 22, 28

Ham, Chris, 166
Haringey PCT, 36, 197
health and social care integration, 108–9
Health Dialog Solutions, 7
Health Foundation, 192
health promotion and ill health
    prevention, 58–9, 74–7, 135
Healthcare Commission (HCC), 190, 191,
    193, 195
HealthPartners, 22, 25–6
Help the Aged, 189, 190
High-impact User Manager (HUM)
    system, 7
high-risk people, identification of, 58–9,
    74–7, 135

Improving Chronic Illness Care (ICIC),
    22, 29
information and technology, for self-care,
    175–9
inspirational leadership, 200
Institute for Clinical Systems
    Improvement, 25
Institute for Healthcare Improvement, 8,
    29, 170
Institute of Public Policy, 110, 113

Integrated Cancer Care Programme
(ICCP), 125–7, 129
and case management, 131–2
integrated models, of social care, 114
interagency and partnership working,
60–61, 77–8
International Alliance of Patient
Organisations, 199
international models, of health care, 22–30

joint NHS, and social care, 36–7

Kaiser Care Management Institute, 24
Kaiser Foundation Hospitals, 24
Kaiser model, 12
Kaiser Permanente, 24–5, 174
King's Fund, 7, 18, 38, 96, 107, 146, 152,
180, 196
Knowledge and Skills Framework (KSF), 44
Knowsley Metropolitan Borough
Council, 36
Knowsley PCT, 36

lay-led self-management processes, 174
leaders
meaning, 145
practitioners as, 156
leadership, 144, 150–52
and advanced practice, 157–8
in long-term conditions, 159–60
arenas for, 151–2
in case management, 154–5
and change, 155–6
competence, levels of, 150
in complex systems, 155
effective leadership, 153
delivering, 145–6
empowerment and influencing, 149–50
in every role, 156–7
issue, 144
meaning, 144–5
NHS, leadership framework in, 146–7
organizations, impact on, 153–4
political understanding and functioning,
148
prescribing, 158
skills in, 147–8
target setting and delivering outcomes,
148–9
long-term conditions, definition of, 1
Luton PCT, 35

managed care models
definition, 19
impact, 21
in United States, 19, 20
management approaches, development
of, 3–4
Manchester PCT, 33–4, 36
McColl Institute for Healthcare
Innovation, 25
Medalink, 178
Mental Capacity Act, 139
models, for self-care, 171–3
Modern Hospice Movement, 123
Modernising Leadership Model, 150
MyGroupHealth, 25

national and international case
management models, 18
case management, data for, 38
England, models in use in, 30–31
evaluation, 38–40
international models, of care, 22
Alaskan Medical Service, 22–3
Amsterdam HealthCare System, 27
Anthem Blue Cross and Blue
Shield, 26
Expanded Chronic Care Model, 29
Green Ribbon Health, 30
Group Health Cooperative, 25
Guided Care, 28
HealthPartners, 25–6
Improving Chronic Illness Care, 29
Kaiser Permanente, 24–5
National model of chronic disease
prevention and control, 28
Outcome intervention model, 28
Pfizer model, 29
Program of All-Inclusive Care for the
Elderly (PACE), 28–9
Touchpoint Health Plan, 26
UnitedHealth Europe Evercare, 26
Veterans Affairs, 29
joint NHS and social care, 36–7
managed care models, impact of, 21
NHS, case management models in,
20–21, 32–6
social care, care management in, 32
national guidelines and evidence-based
practice, for case management
models, 8

National Health Service (NHS), 1, 12, 14,
    18, 44, 105, 164, 180, 185
  cancer plan, 124, 140
  case management in, 11–13, 20–21, 32–6
  case management models, for long-term
      conditions, 1, 11–13
    chronic conditions, management
      of, 9–10
    chronic disease, impact and
      cost of, 6–7
    developing case management and
      care delivery, 4–5, 10–11
    embedding evidence in practice, 8–9
    health care, future of, 5–6
    identification of patients in need of,
      7–8
    management approaches,
      development of, 3–4
    modernising care in, 10
    national guidelines and
      evidence-based practice, 8
    partnerships and expectations, 13–15
    primary care management, 2–3
    self-management and self-care,
      promotion of, 13
  key facets, 30–31
  modernising care in, 10
  need for, 185
National Institute for Health and Clinical
    Excellence (NICE), 5, 173, 174–5
National model of chronic disease
    prevention and control, 28
National Nursing Research Unit, 156
National Prescribing Centre, 158
National Primary Care Collaborative, 3
National Primary Care Research and
    Development Centre, 172
National Service Frameworks (NSFs), 2,
    30, 105, 106, 182, 188, 196
National Workforce Projects, 45
New York Centre for Health and Public
    Service Research, 7
New Zealand model, 28
Next Stage Review, 10
NHS Centre for Reviews and
    Dissemination, 5
NHS Choices, 178
NHS Constitution, 55
NHS Direct Online, 178
NHS Leadership Framework, 144, 146–7,
    152

NHS Modernisation Agency, 20, 44
NHS White Paper, 14, 175
Nursing and Midwifery Council (NMC),
    45, 78, 157, 158

older people and social care, outcomes of
    case management for, 105, 118–19
  commissioning of services, 111–12
  cost of care for, 109–11
  health and social care integration, 108–9
  impact, 114–18
  integrated models of care, 114
  managing resources, 118
  needs and expectations, 111–12
  offerings, 112–13
  policy drivers for care, 105–8
organisational leaders, 145
organisational leadership, 144
outcome intervention model, 28

palliative care, definition of, 123–4
partnerships
  and expectations
    of care delivery, 13–15
  with patients and carers, 199–200
  requirement, 199
patient experience, and outcomes of care,
    195–6
patient-centred health care, 194, 195
Patients at Risk of Re-hospitalisation
    (PARR) tool, 7, 35
patients/service users, outcomes on
  advanced clinical nursing practice, 85–91
  cancer care and end-of-life care, 123
    advanced care planning, 139–40
    case management and ICCP, 131–2
    case management competencies,
      132–7
    competencies, need for, 137–8
    delivering choice programmes, 140
    delivering pilots, 129
    Gold Standards Framework (GSF), for
      palliative care, 125
    Integrated Cancer Care Programme
      (ICCP), 125–7
    pilot programmes, preparing for,
      127–9
    preferred place of care, 140
    programme outcomes, 130–31
  complex care management, 66
    case studies, 78–82

competence and deliverables, 66–74
high-risk patients identification,
   health promotion and ill health
   prevention, 74–7
interagency and partnership working,
   77–8
end of life, managing care at, 97–101
expectations from care, 186–7
experience, 190–92, 195
   assessments, 192–4
   in case management, 197–9
government expectations, 186
improvements, 188–90
modernisation for, 188
outcomes of care and patient experience,
   195–6
partnerships, with patients and carers,
   199–200
patient-centred care, 195
proactively manage complex long-term
   conditions, 91–4
professional practice and leadership,
   94–7
provision of information on, 201
Public Service Agreement (PSA)
   targets, 192
quality for, 200–201
reported outcomes, from management
   of long-term conditions, 187–8
requirements, 186–7
and self-care
   engaging patients in, 179–80
   evidence base, 173–5
   Expert Patient Programme (EPP),
      168–9
   meaning, 164–7
   models, 171–3
   practitioners, and self-care, 167–8
   programmes, 169–70
   staff role, 170–71
   systems for, 168
   using information and technology,
      175–9
Permanente Medical Groups, 24
Pfizer model, 29
Picker Institute, 130, 193
pilot programmes, 114
   delivering, 129
   development, 126–7
   evaluations, 130
   implementation, 130–31

preparing for, 127–9
   risk stratification, 131–2
practitioners
   as leaders, 156
   and self-care, 167–8
'preferred place of care', 140
primary care
   developing and delivering care, 4–5
   future, 5–6
   long-term conditions, management
      of, 2–3
   in United Kingdom, 19
Primary Care Contracting, 173
primary care trusts (PCTs), 1, 18, 33, 34,
   35, 169
proactively manage complex long-term
   conditions, 91–4, 134
professional practice and leadership,
   57–8, 94–7
Program of All-Inclusive Care for the
   Elderly (PACE) model, 28–9
PSA Delivery Agreement 19, 192
Public Service Agreement (PSA) target,
   12, 192

Quality and Outcomes Framework, 2, 3
   in primary care, 9–10

reactive palliation, 124
reason for implementation, of case
   management for long-term
   conditions, 185
Richards, Mike, 141
risk stratification, in case management,
   131–2
Royal College of Nursing (RCN), 43–4
Royal Pharmaceutical Society of Great
   Britain, 158

Salford NHS Hospitals Trust, 172
Saunders, Cicely, 123
self-belief, 146–7
self-care, 55–6
   engaging patients in, 179–80
   evidence base, 173–5
   Expert Patient Programme (EPP), 168–9
   meaning, 164–7
   models, 171–3
   and patient outcomes, 164
   and practitioners, 167–8
   programmes, 169–70

self-care (*Continued*)
  and self-management, 135, 166
  staff role, 170–71
  systems for, 168
  using information and technology for,
    175–9
'Self Care for Primary Care Professionals
    Project', 172
self-management, 55–6
  definition, 166
  and self-care, 13
service integration, 114
Skills for Health, 44
social care, 185, 194
  care management in, 32
  joint NHS and, 36–7
staff role, for promoting self-care,
    170–71
Strategic Health Authority (SHA), 33, 62
Strategic Nursing Leaders programme, 152

Touchpoint Health Plan, 26
transactional leadership, 153
transformational leadership, 153

United HealthCare, 31, 33, 130
United Kingdom, primary care model in,
    19
United States
  chronic care model, 20
  healthcare system, 19, 20
  managed care in, 19
UnitedHealth Europe, 26, 125, 127, 141
UnitedHealth Group, 11
unpaid carers, 110
US healthcare environment, 18, 19, 20

Veterans Affairs, 29

Wanless, Derek, 5, 107
Wanless Social Care Review, 107, 196
Warrington PCT, 36
'Working in Partnership Programme',
    172
World Health Organisation, 7, 43, 123